CONTENTS

Chapter 1: Introduction to Chiari Malformation — 1

Chapter 2: Anatomy and Physiology of the Central Nervous System — 7

Chapter 3: Pathophysiology of Chiari Malformation — 19

Chapter 4: Clinical Presentation and Diagnosis — 32

Chapter 5: Management Strategies — 46

Chapter 6: Complications and Prognosis — 63

Chapter 7: Research Advances and Future Directions — 77

Chapter 8: Holistic Approaches to Chiari Malformation Management — 89

CHAPTER 1: INTRODUCTION TO CHIARI MALFORMATION

Definition and Classification of Chiari Malformation

Chiari malformation, named after the Austrian pathologist Hans Chiari who first described it in the late 19th century, is a structural abnormality of the brain characterized by the downward displacement of the cerebellar tonsils through the foramen magnum (the large opening at the base of the skull). This displacement can lead to compression of the brainstem and blockage of normal cerebrospinal fluid (CSF) circulation, resulting in a range of neurological symptoms. Chiari malformation is classified into several types based on the severity of the anatomical abnormalities and the presence of associated features.

Types of Chiari Malformation:

1. **Chiari Malformation Type I (CM-I):**
   - CM-I is the most common form and typically manifests during childhood or adolescence.
   - It is characterized by the downward displacement of the cerebellar tonsils below the foramen magnum, without involvement of the brainstem.
   - This type is often asymptomatic but can present

with symptoms such as headaches, neck pain, dizziness, and sensory disturbances.

2. **Chiari Malformation Type II (CM-II):**
   - CM-II is usually associated with myelomeningocele, a form of spina bifida, and occurs in infancy.
   - In addition to cerebellar tonsillar herniation, there is also caudal displacement of the brainstem and fourth ventricle.
   - Patients with CM-II often have more severe neurological deficits, including hydrocephalus and paralysis of the lower extremities.

3. **Chiari Malformation Type III (CM-III):**
   - CM-III is the rarest and most severe form, characterized by extensive herniation of the cerebellum and brainstem through a defect in the posterior fossa.
   - This type is associated with significant neurological deficits and is often incompatible with life.

4. **Chiari Malformation Type IV (CM-IV):**
   - CM-IV is characterized by cerebellar hypoplasia or aplasia, where the cerebellum fails to develop properly.
   - This type is extremely rare and can be associated with other structural brain abnormalities.

Additional Classifications:

In addition to the anatomical classification, Chiari malformation can also be classified based on the presence of associated conditions or secondary features:

1. **Syringomyelia:** Some individuals with Chiari malformation may develop syringomyelia, a condition characterized by the formation of fluid-filled cavities within the spinal cord. This can lead to progressive neurological symptoms such as weakness, sensory loss,

and bladder dysfunction.
2. **Hydrocephalus:** Compression of the brainstem and obstruction of CSF flow in Chiari malformation can lead to the development of hydrocephalus, a condition characterized by the accumulation of CSF within the brain ventricles. Hydrocephalus can exacerbate neurological symptoms and may require surgical intervention.
3. **Tethered Cord Syndrome:** In some cases, Chiari malformation may be associated with tethered cord syndrome, where the spinal cord is abnormally attached to surrounding tissues. This can result in stretching of the spinal cord and compression of nerve roots, leading to symptoms such as back pain, leg weakness, and bladder dysfunction.
4. **Associated Skeletal Anomalies:** Chiari malformation may occur in conjunction with other skeletal anomalies, such as basilar invagination (a condition where the upper cervical vertebrae protrude into the skull base), craniosynostosis (premature fusion of skull bones), or Klippel-Feil syndrome (congenital fusion of cervical vertebrae).

In summary, Chiari malformation encompasses a spectrum of structural abnormalities of the brain and skull base, with varying degrees of severity and associated features. Understanding the classification and associated conditions is crucial for accurate diagnosis, treatment planning, and prognostication in individuals affected by this complex neurological disorder.

Etiology and Risk Factors of Chiari Malformation

Chiari malformation is a complex neurological disorder characterized by the downward displacement of the cerebellar tonsils through the foramen magnum, leading to compression of the brainstem and disruption of normal cerebrospinal fluid (CSF) dynamics. While the precise etiology of Chiari malformation remains incompletely understood, it is believed to involve a combination of genetic, developmental, and environmental factors. In this section, we explore the current understanding of the etiology and potential risk factors associated with Chiari malformation.

Genetic Factors:

There is growing evidence to suggest a genetic predisposition to Chiari malformation, with familial clustering observed in some cases. Studies have identified several genetic mutations and chromosomal abnormalities associated with Chiari malformation, implicating multiple genes involved in craniofacial and neural development. Notably, mutations in genes encoding proteins involved in the formation of the posterior cranial fossa, such as the homeobox gene *PAX1* and the transcription factor *ZIC1*, have been implicated in the pathogenesis of Chiari malformation. Additionally, variations in genes related to extracellular matrix remodeling, neurogenesis, and neuronal migration have also been implicated in the development of Chiari malformation.

Developmental Factors:

Chiari malformation is thought to arise from abnormalities in the development of the posterior cranial fossa during embryogenesis. The posterior cranial fossa is formed by the occipital bone and plays a crucial role in housing and protecting the brainstem and cerebellum. Disruptions in the intricate process of skull and brain development during fetal development can lead to inadequate space within the posterior cranial fossa, predisposing individuals to Chiari malformation. Factors such as abnormal growth of the skull bones, cranial base abnormalities, and impaired cerebellar development have been implicated in the pathogenesis of Chiari malformation.

Environmental Factors:

While genetic and developmental factors play a significant role in the pathogenesis of Chiari malformation, environmental factors may also contribute to its development. Maternal exposure to certain teratogenic agents or environmental toxins during pregnancy has been proposed as potential risk factors for Chiari malformation. Additionally, intrauterine factors such as oligohydramnios (reduced amniotic fluid volume) or uterine constraints may impact fetal skull and brain development, increasing the risk of Chiari malformation.

Cranial Base Abnormalities:

Abnormalities in the structure and morphology of the cranial base have been implicated in the pathogenesis of Chiari malformation. Conditions such as basilar invagination, where the upper cervical vertebrae protrude into the skull base, can reduce the volume of the posterior cranial fossa and exacerbate cerebellar herniation. Craniosynostosis, a condition characterized by premature fusion of skull bones, can also alter the shape and size of the cranial base, predisposing individuals to Chiari malformation.

Connective Tissue Disorders:

Chiari malformation is frequently associated with connective tissue disorders such as Ehlers-Danlos syndrome and Marfan syndrome. These conditions are characterized by abnormalities in the structure and function of collagen and other extracellular matrix components, leading to laxity and weakness of connective tissues throughout the body. Connective tissue abnormalities may contribute to the development of Chiari malformation by altering the biomechanical properties of the skull and spinal canal, predisposing individuals to cerebellar herniation.

Other Risk Factors:

Several other factors have been proposed as potential risk factors for Chiari malformation, although their role remains less well-established. These include maternal diabetes mellitus, maternal obesity, maternal smoking during pregnancy, and certain medications or drug exposures during fetal development. Further research is needed to elucidate the specific contributions of these factors to the pathogenesis of Chiari malformation.

In conclusion, Chiari malformation is a complex disorder with multifactorial etiology involving genetic, developmental, and environmental factors. Understanding the interplay between these factors is crucial for elucidating the pathogenesis of Chiari malformation and may ultimately lead to the development of novel therapeutic strategies and preventive measures. Further research is warranted to unravel the intricate mechanisms underlying this intriguing neurological condition.

CHAPTER 2: ANATOMY AND PHYSIOLOGY OF THE CENTRAL NERVOUS SYSTEM

Overview of the Central Nervous System

The central nervous system (CNS) serves as the command center of the human body, orchestrating a vast array of sensory, motor, and cognitive functions essential for survival and well-being. Comprising the brain and spinal cord, the CNS plays a fundamental role in processing information, coordinating movements, regulating bodily functions, and generating consciousness. In this section, we provide a comprehensive overview of the structure, organization, and functions of the central nervous system.

Anatomy of the Brain:

The brain, the most complex organ in the human body, is divided into several distinct regions, each with specialized functions. The major divisions of the brain include the cerebrum, cerebellum, and brainstem.

1. **Cerebrum:** Occupying the largest portion of the brain, the cerebrum is responsible for higher cognitive functions such as perception, thought, memory, and voluntary movement. It is divided into two hemispheres, each further subdivided into lobes. The frontal lobe controls motor functions, executive functions, and personality, while the parietal lobe processes sensory information such as touch and spatial awareness. The temporal lobe is involved in auditory processing and memory, while the occipital lobe is dedicated to visual processing.
2. **Cerebellum:** Situated beneath the cerebrum, the cerebellum is primarily responsible for coordinating motor movements, maintaining balance, and posture. Despite its smaller size compared to the cerebrum, the cerebellum contains a highly convoluted surface with intricate neural circuits crucial for motor coordination and learning.
3. **Brainstem:** The brainstem, located at the base of the brain, serves as a critical relay center connecting the brain to the spinal cord. It consists of three main regions: the midbrain, pons, and medulla oblongata. The brainstem regulates essential functions such as breathing, heart rate, blood pressure, and consciousness. It also serves as the gateway for sensory and motor pathways traveling between the brain and spinal cord.

Anatomy of the Spinal Cord:

The spinal cord, a cylindrical bundle of nerve fibers enclosed within the vertebral column, acts as a conduit for communication between the brain and peripheral nervous system. It is organized into segments corresponding to different regions of the body and is surrounded by protective layers of connective tissue known as the meninges. The spinal cord contains both ascending sensory pathways, which transmit sensory information from the body to the brain, and descending motor pathways, which convey motor commands from the brain to the muscles and glands.

Cerebrospinal Fluid Dynamics:

Cerebrospinal fluid (CSF) is a clear, colorless fluid that fills the ventricles of the brain and the subarachnoid space surrounding the brain and spinal cord. Produced by specialized structures called choroid plexuses within the brain ventricles, CSF serves several crucial functions. It acts as a cushion, protecting the brain and spinal cord from mechanical shocks and trauma. CSF also helps maintain a stable extracellular environment within the CNS by transporting nutrients, removing waste products, and regulating intracranial pressure. Additionally, CSF circulation plays a vital role in maintaining homeostasis and facilitating the exchange of biochemical signals within the CNS.

Neurovascular Anatomy:

The central nervous system is highly vascularized, with a rich network of blood vessels supplying oxygen and nutrients to brain tissue. The cerebral circulation is composed of two main arterial systems: the anterior circulation, supplied by the internal carotid arteries, and the posterior circulation, supplied by the vertebral arteries. These arterial systems converge to form the Circle of Willis, a critical vascular structure located at the base of the brain that ensures adequate blood supply to the brain's various regions. Disruptions in cerebral blood flow can lead to ischemic stroke, hemorrhagic stroke, or other cerebrovascular disorders with potentially devastating consequences.

In summary, the central nervous system is a marvel of biological engineering, comprising intricate neural networks and vascular structures essential for human cognition, movement, and homeostasis. Understanding the anatomy and physiology of the CNS is fundamental for elucidating the mechanisms underlying neurological disorders and developing effective therapeutic interventions to preserve and restore brain function.

Anatomy of the Brainstem and Cerebellum

The brainstem and cerebellum are vital structures located at the base of the brain, playing crucial roles in coordinating motor functions, regulating vital autonomic processes, and facilitating sensory integration. Despite their relatively small size compared to the cerebrum, these regions exhibit remarkable complexity and are essential for maintaining overall brain function. In this section, we delve into the anatomy and functional significance of the brainstem and cerebellum.

Anatomy of the Brainstem:

The brainstem serves as a bridge between the brain and spinal cord, housing nuclei responsible for essential autonomic and motor functions. It consists of three main regions: the midbrain, pons, and medulla oblongata.

1. **Midbrain (Mesencephalon):** Situated between the diencephalon and the pons, the midbrain serves as a relay center for visual, auditory, and motor pathways. It contains nuclei involved in the regulation of eye movements, including the superior colliculi (responsible for visual reflexes) and the oculomotor nucleus (responsible for controlling eye movements). Additionally, the midbrain houses the substantia nigra, a dopaminergic structure involved in motor control and implicated in Parkinson's disease.
2. **Pons:** The pons lies anterior to the cerebellum and serves as a conduit for information traveling between the cerebrum, cerebellum, and spinal cord. It contains nuclei involved in regulating respiration, sleep-wake cycles, and cranial nerve functions. Notably, the pontine nuclei relay motor signals from the cerebral cortex

to the cerebellum via the middle cerebellar peduncles, facilitating coordination and motor learning.
3. **Medulla Oblongata:** The medulla oblongata, located below the pons, is responsible for regulating vital autonomic functions such as heart rate, blood pressure, breathing, and swallowing. It contains nuclei controlling respiratory rhythm generation, including the dorsal respiratory group (involved in inspiration) and the ventral respiratory group (involved in expiration). Additionally, the medulla houses vital centers for cardiovascular control, such as the vasomotor center and the cardiac center.

Anatomy of the Cerebellum:

The cerebellum, situated dorsal to the brainstem, is essential for coordinating voluntary movements, maintaining balance, and modulating motor learning and cognition. Despite its relatively small size, the cerebellum contains more neurons than the rest of the brain combined, underscoring its importance in motor control and coordination.

1. **Cerebellar Cortex:** The outer layer of the cerebellum, known as the cerebellar cortex, is highly convoluted and contains numerous folia (folds) and fissures. It is organized into three distinct layers: the molecular layer, the Purkinje cell layer, and the granular layer. The cerebellar cortex receives input from the brainstem and cerebral cortex via mossy fibers and climbing fibers, respectively, and integrates this information to regulate motor output.
2. **Deep Cerebellar Nuclei:** Located deep within the cerebellum, the deep cerebellar nuclei consist of four main nuclei: the dentate nucleus, interposed nuclei (comprising the globose and emboliform nuclei), and the fastigial nucleus. These nuclei serve as the output centers of the cerebellum, transmitting processed motor signals to the brainstem and thalamus for further processing and

integration.
3. **Cerebellar Peduncles:** The cerebellum is connected to the brainstem via three pairs of fiber bundles known as cerebellar peduncles: the superior cerebellar peduncles, the middle cerebellar peduncles, and the inferior cerebellar peduncles. These peduncles facilitate bidirectional communication between the cerebellum and other brain regions, allowing for the coordination of motor activities and the maintenance of posture and balance.

Functional Significance:

The brainstem and cerebellum play complementary roles in regulating motor functions and maintaining homeostasis within the central nervous system. While the brainstem is primarily involved in vital autonomic processes such as respiration, cardiovascular control, and cranial nerve functions, the cerebellum specializes in fine-tuning voluntary movements, coordinating muscle activity, and adapting motor responses to changing environmental demands. Dysfunction of the brainstem or cerebellum can lead to a range of neurological deficits, including motor impairment, gait disturbances, and autonomic dysfunction, underscoring the critical importance of these structures in human health and well-being.

In conclusion, the brainstem and cerebellum represent essential components of the central nervous system, playing pivotal roles in regulating motor coordination, maintaining balance, and ensuring the smooth execution of voluntary movements. Understanding the intricate anatomy and functional organization of these regions is crucial for elucidating the pathophysiology of neurological disorders and developing targeted therapeutic interventions to restore brain function and improve patient outcomes.

Cerebrospinal Fluid Dynamics

Cerebrospinal fluid (CSF) is a clear, colorless fluid that fills the ventricles of the brain and the subarachnoid space surrounding the brain and spinal cord. It serves several crucial functions within the central nervous system (CNS), including cushioning and protecting the brain and spinal cord from mechanical shocks, providing buoyancy to support the weight of the brain, and facilitating the exchange of nutrients and waste products between the CNS and systemic circulation. In this section, we explore the dynamics of CSF circulation, including its production, circulation, and absorption, and its role in maintaining CNS homeostasis.

Production of Cerebrospinal Fluid:

CSF is primarily produced by specialized structures within the brain known as choroid plexuses, which are located in the walls of the brain ventricles. The choroid plexus consists of a highly vascularized network of capillaries enclosed by a layer of epithelial cells. These epithelial cells actively transport ions and other solutes from the blood into the ventricles, creating an osmotic gradient that drives the movement of water into the ventricles, ultimately leading to CSF formation. The composition of CSF is similar to that of plasma, albeit with lower protein and glucose concentrations and higher concentrations of certain ions such as sodium and chloride.

Circulation of Cerebrospinal Fluid:

Once formed, CSF circulates within the ventricular system of the brain and the subarachnoid space surrounding the brain and spinal cord. CSF flow is facilitated by the beating of cilia on the ependymal cells lining the ventricles, which generate rhythmic movements that propel CSF through the ventricular system. CSF flows from the lateral ventricles into the third ventricle via the interventricular foramina (foramina of Monro), then into the fourth ventricle via the cerebral aqueduct (aqueduct of Sylvius). From the fourth ventricle, CSF exits the ventricular system and enters the subarachnoid space through three openings: the median aperture (foramen of Magendie) and the two lateral apertures (foramina of Luschka).

Within the subarachnoid space, CSF circulates around the brain and spinal cord, bathing these structures in a protective fluid layer. CSF flow within the subarachnoid space is driven by a combination of pulsatile movements of blood vessels and the rhythmic expansion and contraction of the brain and spinal cord during the cardiac and respiratory cycles. This dynamic flow pattern helps to distribute CSF throughout the CNS, ensuring uniform support and protection of neural tissues.

Absorption of Cerebrospinal Fluid:

CSF is primarily absorbed into the bloodstream via specialized structures known as arachnoid villi or granulations, located within the subarachnoid space. Arachnoid villi are protrusions of the arachnoid membrane that extend into the dural sinuses, large venous channels located between the layers of the dura mater that surround the brain. CSF is absorbed into the bloodstream across the thin walls of the arachnoid villi, where it mixes with venous blood and is subsequently carried away from the brain and spinal cord.

In addition to arachnoid villi, recent studies have identified alternative pathways for CSF absorption, including drainage through lymphatic vessels located within the meninges and along cranial nerves. These lymphatic pathways provide an additional route for CSF clearance from the CNS and may play a role in the pathophysiology of neurodegenerative diseases and CNS disorders.

Regulation of Cerebrospinal Fluid Dynamics:

The production, circulation, and absorption of CSF are tightly regulated processes that maintain the delicate balance of fluid volume and pressure within the CNS. Several mechanisms contribute to the regulation of CSF dynamics, including the production and secretion of CSF by the choroid plexus, the compliance and elasticity of the brain and spinal cord, and the pressure differentials between CSF and blood. Disruption of CSF dynamics can lead to alterations in intracranial pressure, hydrocephalus (accumulation of CSF within the brain ventricles), or other CNS disorders.

In summary, cerebrospinal fluid dynamics play a critical role in maintaining CNS homeostasis and ensuring the optimal functioning of neural tissues. Understanding the mechanisms underlying CSF production, circulation, and absorption is essential for elucidating the pathophysiology of neurological disorders and developing targeted therapies to restore CSF dynamics and improve patient outcomes. Further research into the regulation of CSF dynamics and its role in CNS health and disease holds promise for advancing our understanding of neurologic conditions and developing novel therapeutic interventions.

Neurovascular Anatomy in Relation to Chiari Malformation

Chiari malformation is a complex neurological disorder characterized by the herniation of cerebellar tonsils through the foramen magnum, leading to compression of the brainstem and disruption of normal cerebrospinal fluid (CSF) dynamics. While the etiology of Chiari malformation is multifactorial, abnormalities in neurovascular anatomy have been implicated in the pathogenesis and progression of this condition. In this section, we explore the intricate interplay between neurovascular structures and Chiari malformation, highlighting the anatomical features and vascular dynamics that contribute to the development and clinical manifestations of this disorder.

Anatomy of the Craniovertebral Junction:

The craniovertebral junction (CVJ) represents the complex anatomical region where the skull base meets the upper cervical spine. This region is critical for maintaining the stability and mobility of the head and neck and is characterized by a series of bony and ligamentous structures that provide support and protection to the neurovascular elements passing through it. Key structures within the CVJ include the occipital bone, atlas (C1), axis (C2), dens (odontoid process), transverse ligament, alar ligaments, and apical ligament. Additionally, the vertebral arteries traverse the CVJ, passing through bony foramina within the cervical vertebrae and contributing to the blood supply of the brainstem and cerebellum.

Implications for Chiari Malformation:

Abnormalities in the anatomy of the CVJ, such as basilar invagination (protrusion of the odontoid process into the foramen magnum) or atlantoaxial instability, can lead to mechanical compression of the brainstem and upper cervical spinal cord, predisposing individuals to Chiari malformation. Basilar invagination, in particular, can reduce the volume of the posterior cranial fossa and impede normal CSF circulation, exacerbating cerebellar herniation and neurological symptoms. Additionally, atlantoaxial instability can result in abnormal movements of the odontoid process, further compromising the integrity of the CVJ and exacerbating Chiari malformation-related symptoms.

Neurovascular Structures:

The neurovascular structures within the CVJ, including the

vertebral arteries and associated venous plexuses, play a critical role in maintaining blood supply to the brainstem and cerebellum. The vertebral arteries, arising from the subclavian arteries, ascend through the transverse foramina of the cervical vertebrae before entering the skull through the foramen magnum. These arteries give rise to the posterior cerebral circulation and contribute to the arterial supply of the brainstem and cerebellum. Additionally, the venous plexuses surrounding the CVJ, including the vertebral venous plexus and suboccipital venous plexus, provide drainage pathways for venous blood from the brain and spinal cord.

Vascular Compression Syndromes:

In some cases of Chiari malformation, vascular compression syndromes may coexist, further exacerbating neurological symptoms and complicating management. Vascular compression syndromes occur when neurovascular structures, such as the vertebral arteries or adjacent venous plexuses, become compressed or compromised by bony or soft tissue abnormalities within the CVJ. This compression can lead to ischemia, hypoperfusion, or venous congestion in the brainstem or cerebellum, resulting in neurological deficits such as vertigo, ataxia, or cranial nerve dysfunction.

Surgical Considerations:

Surgical management of Chiari malformation often involves decompression of the CVJ to relieve pressure on the brainstem and restore normal CSF dynamics. Surgical techniques may include suboccipital craniectomy, resection of the posterior arch of the atlas, or stabilization of the CVJ with instrumentation. However, careful consideration must be given to the preservation of neurovascular structures during surgical intervention to minimize the risk of vascular injury or complications. Preoperative imaging studies, such as magnetic resonance angiography (MRA) or computed tomography angiography (CTA), are essential for assessing vascular anatomy and planning surgical approaches.

Conclusion:

Neurovascular anatomy plays a significant role in the pathogenesis and clinical manifestations of Chiari malformation. Abnormalities within the CVJ can lead to mechanical compression of the brainstem and upper cervical spinal cord, exacerbating cerebellar herniation and neurological symptoms. Additionally, vascular compression syndromes may coexist, further complicating management and necessitating careful consideration of surgical approaches. Understanding the intricate interplay between neurovascular structures and Chiari malformation is essential for optimizing patient care and improving outcomes in individuals affected by this complex neurological disorder. Further research into the underlying mechanisms and therapeutic interventions targeting neurovascular anatomy holds promise for advancing our understanding and management of Chiari malformation in clinical practice.

CHAPTER 3: PATHOPHYSIOLOGY OF CHIARI MALFORMATION

Mechanisms of Malformation Development in Chiari Malformation

Chiari malformation is a complex neurological disorder characterized by the downward displacement of the cerebellar tonsils through the foramen magnum, leading to compression of the brainstem and disruption of normal cerebrospinal fluid (CSF) dynamics. While the exact mechanisms underlying the development of Chiari malformation remain incompletely understood, several factors, including genetic predisposition, abnormal craniovertebral anatomy, and altered CSF dynamics, have been implicated in its pathogenesis. In this section, we explore the various mechanisms proposed to contribute to the development and progression of Chiari malformation, shedding light on the intricate interplay between genetic, developmental, and biomechanical factors.

Genetic Predisposition:

There is growing evidence to suggest a genetic component to the development of Chiari malformation, with familial clustering observed in some cases. Genome-wide association studies (GWAS) and genetic linkage analyses have identified several candidate genes and chromosomal loci associated with Chiari malformation, implicating multiple genetic pathways involved in craniofacial and neural development. Mutations in genes encoding proteins crucial for the formation of the posterior cranial fossa, such as *PAX1* and *ZIC1*, have been identified in individuals with Chiari malformation, highlighting the importance of genetic factors in predisposing individuals to this condition. Additionally, variations in genes involved in extracellular matrix remodeling, neurogenesis, and neuronal migration have also been implicated in the pathogenesis of Chiari malformation, underscoring the multifactorial nature of this disorder.

Abnormal Craniovertebral Anatomy:

Alterations in the anatomy of the craniovertebral junction (CVJ), where the skull base meets the upper cervical spine, have been implicated in the development of Chiari malformation. Basilar invagination, characterized by the protrusion of the odontoid process into the foramen magnum, can reduce the volume of the posterior cranial fossa and impede normal CSF circulation, predisposing individuals to cerebellar herniation. Similarly, atlantoaxial instability, resulting from laxity or malformation of ligaments supporting the CVJ, can lead to abnormal movements of the odontoid process and compromise the integrity of the foramen magnum, further exacerbating Chiari malformation-related symptoms. Additionally, abnormalities in the shape and size of the posterior cranial fossa, such as reduced volume or increased slope, have been associated with an increased risk of Chiari malformation, highlighting the importance of craniovertebral anatomy in the pathogenesis of this disorder.

Altered Cerebrospinal Fluid Dynamics:

Disruptions in normal cerebrospinal fluid (CSF) dynamics have long been implicated in the pathogenesis of Chiari malformation. CSF plays a crucial role in maintaining the buoyancy and stability of the brain within the cranial vault and facilitating the exchange of nutrients and waste products between the brain and systemic circulation. Abnormalities in CSF production, circulation, or absorption can lead to alterations in intracranial pressure and CSF hydrodynamics, predisposing individuals to cerebellar herniation and Chiari malformation. For example, conditions that increase CSF production or impair CSF absorption, such as hydrocephalus or venous outflow obstruction, can lead to elevated intracranial pressure and exacerbate Chiari malformation-related symptoms. Similarly, disruptions in CSF flow dynamics within the subarachnoid space, such as arachnoid cysts or syringomyelia, can create focal areas of pressure gradients and further impede normal CSF circulation, contributing to the pathogenesis of Chiari malformation.

Biomechanical Factors:

Biomechanical factors, including altered tissue elasticity, tensile strength, and viscoelastic properties, may also play a role in the development of Chiari malformation. Abnormalities in connective tissue structure and composition, such as collagen or elastin defects, can lead to laxity or weakness of ligaments supporting the CVJ, predisposing individuals to atlantoaxial instability and craniovertebral malformations. Additionally, alterations in cranial vault shape or craniospinal compliance may affect the distribution and transmission of intracranial pressure, further exacerbating the downward displacement of cerebellar structures and contributing to the pathogenesis of Chiari malformation.

In conclusion, Chiari malformation represents a complex

interplay of genetic, developmental, and biomechanical factors that collectively contribute to the downward displacement of cerebellar structures and disruption of normal CNS function. Understanding the underlying mechanisms of Chiari malformation is crucial for elucidating its pathogenesis and guiding therapeutic interventions aimed at alleviating symptoms and improving patient outcomes. Further research into the genetic and molecular pathways involved in Chiari malformation holds promise for advancing our understanding of this condition and developing targeted therapies to address its underlying causes.

Impact on Cerebrospinal Fluid Circulation in Chiari Malformation

Chiari malformation is a complex neurological disorder characterized by the downward displacement of the cerebellar tonsils through the foramen magnum, leading to compression of the brainstem and disruption of normal cerebrospinal fluid (CSF) dynamics. The abnormal anatomy and structural changes associated with Chiari malformation can have profound effects on CSF circulation, leading to alterations in intracranial pressure, impaired CSF flow dynamics, and the development of secondary complications such as syringomyelia. In this section, we explore the impact of Chiari malformation on CSF circulation and the mechanisms underlying its pathophysiology.

Compression of CSF Pathways:

The primary mechanism by which Chiari malformation affects CSF circulation is through mechanical compression of CSF pathways at the level of the foramen magnum. The downward displacement of the cerebellar tonsils can obstruct the normal flow of CSF through the cerebral aqueduct, fourth ventricle, and subarachnoid space, leading to impaired CSF circulation and elevated intracranial pressure. Additionally, compression of the brainstem can further impede CSF flow dynamics, exacerbating the accumulation of fluid within the ventricular system and contributing to the development of hydrocephalus.

Obstruction of CSF Absorption:

In addition to mechanical compression of CSF pathways, Chiari malformation can also impair the absorption of CSF into the venous circulation, further exacerbating disturbances in CSF dynamics. Compression of the arachnoid villi or granulations within the subarachnoid space can hinder the normal drainage of CSF into the venous sinuses, leading to elevated intracranial pressure and the formation of periventricular edema. Furthermore, alterations in venous outflow dynamics, such as venous congestion or stenosis, can further impair CSF absorption and contribute to the progression of Chiari malformation-related symptoms.

Alterations in CSF Pressure Gradients:

The displacement of cerebellar structures and compression of CSF pathways in Chiari malformation can disrupt normal CSF pressure gradients within the cranial vault, leading to focal areas of elevated pressure and decreased flow. These pressure differentials can result in the formation of syringomyelia, a condition characterized by the development of fluid-filled cavities within the spinal cord. The exact mechanisms underlying syrinx formation in Chiari malformation remain incompletely understood but are thought to involve alterations in CSF flow dynamics, tissue compliance, and biomechanical factors. Syringomyelia can further exacerbate neurological symptoms and complicate management, underscoring the importance of understanding its pathophysiology in the context of Chiari malformation.

Impact on Brain Compliance and Perfusion:

The disruption of normal CSF circulation in Chiari malformation can also affect brain compliance and perfusion, leading to alterations in cerebral blood flow and metabolic function. Elevated intracranial pressure and impaired CSF absorption can reduce brain compliance and impair the brain's ability to accommodate changes in volume, leading to tissue compression and ischemia. Additionally, alterations in CSF dynamics can disrupt the exchange of nutrients and waste products within the CNS, further compromising neuronal function and viability. These hemodynamic disturbances can contribute to the development of neurological symptoms such as headache, dizziness, cognitive impairment, and motor dysfunction in individuals with Chiari malformation.

Therapeutic Implications:

Understanding the impact of Chiari malformation on CSF circulation is essential for guiding therapeutic interventions aimed at alleviating symptoms and improving patient outcomes. Surgical decompression of the foramen magnum and posterior fossa is the primary treatment modality for Chiari malformation, aimed at relieving mechanical compression of CSF pathways and restoring normal CSF dynamics. Surgical techniques may include suboccipital craniectomy, resection of the posterior arch of the atlas, or duraplasty to expand the posterior fossa and facilitate CSF flow. Additionally, careful monitoring of intracranial pressure and CSF dynamics is essential for optimizing surgical outcomes and minimizing the risk of complications such as hydrocephalus or syringomyelia.

In conclusion, Chiari malformation has profound effects on CSF circulation, leading to alterations in intracranial pressure, impaired CSF flow dynamics, and the development of secondary complications such as syringomyelia. Understanding the mechanisms underlying these disturbances is crucial for guiding therapeutic interventions and improving patient outcomes in individuals affected by this complex neurological disorder. Further research into the pathophysiology of Chiari malformation-related CSF circulation abnormalities holds promise for advancing our understanding of this condition and developing targeted therapies to address its underlying causes.

Compression Effects on Neural Structures in Chiari Malformation

Chiari malformation is a neurological condition characterized by the downward displacement of the cerebellar tonsils through the foramen magnum, resulting in compression of neural structures within the posterior cranial fossa. This compression can lead to a wide range of neurological symptoms and complications, including headache, cranial nerve dysfunction, motor impairment, and syringomyelia. In this section, we explore the effects of compression on neural structures in Chiari malformation, shedding light on the underlying mechanisms and clinical manifestations of this condition.

Compression of the Brainstem:

One of the primary consequences of Chiari malformation is compression of the brainstem, the crucial pathway connecting the brain to the spinal cord and coordinating vital functions such as respiration, heart rate, and consciousness. The downward displacement of the cerebellar tonsils can compress the brainstem against the clivus and upper cervical spinal cord, leading to neurological deficits such as dysphagia, dysarthria, and respiratory disturbances. Compression of the brainstem can also impair the transmission of sensory and motor signals between the brain and peripheral nerves, resulting in sensory deficits, muscle weakness, and coordination difficulties.

Impingement on Cranial Nerves:

The compression of neural structures in Chiari malformation can also affect the function of cranial nerves, leading to a variety of cranial nerve deficits. The lower cranial nerves, including the glossopharyngeal nerve (CN IX), vagus nerve (CN X), and accessory nerve (CN XI), are particularly vulnerable to compression due to their close proximity to the foramen magnum. Compression of these nerves can result in symptoms such as difficulty swallowing (dysphagia), voice changes, hoarseness, and weakness of the shoulder and neck muscles. Additionally, compression of the trigeminal nerve (CN V) may lead to facial pain, numbness, and sensory disturbances.

Cerebellar Dysfunction:

The compression of the cerebellum in Chiari malformation can impair its normal function, leading to deficits in motor coordination, balance, and fine motor control. The cerebellum plays a crucial role in regulating voluntary movements and coordinating muscle activity, and compression-induced dysfunction can result in symptoms such as ataxia (unsteady gait), tremors, and difficulties with fine motor tasks. Additionally, compression of the cerebellum can disrupt the integration of sensory information from the vestibular system and proprioceptors, further exacerbating balance and coordination deficits.

Syringomyelia Formation:

Compression of neural structures in Chiari malformation can also lead to the formation of syringomyelia, a condition characterized by the development of fluid-filled cavities (syrinxes) within the spinal cord. The exact mechanisms underlying syrinx formation in Chiari malformation remain incompletely understood but are thought to involve alterations in cerebrospinal fluid dynamics, tissue compliance, and pressure gradients within the spinal cord. Syringomyelia can further exacerbate neurological symptoms and complicate management, leading to sensory deficits, motor weakness, and autonomic dysfunction.

Hydrocephalus and Intracranial Hypertension:

Compression of the ventricular system and alterations in cerebrospinal fluid dynamics in Chiari malformation can lead to the development of hydrocephalus, a condition characterized by the accumulation of excess CSF within the brain ventricles. Hydrocephalus can further exacerbate intracranial hypertension and compressive effects on neural structures, leading to worsening neurological symptoms and cognitive impairment. Additionally, elevated intracranial pressure can impair cerebral blood flow and metabolic function, further compromising neuronal viability and function.

Clinical Manifestations and Diagnostic Considerations:

The compression effects on neural structures in Chiari malformation manifest clinically as a spectrum of neurological symptoms, including headache, neck pain, dizziness, sensory disturbances, motor weakness, and autonomic dysfunction. Diagnosis of Chiari malformation typically involves a combination of clinical evaluation, neuroimaging studies (such as magnetic resonance imaging), and assessment of CSF dynamics. Management strategies may include surgical decompression of the foramen magnum and posterior fossa, aimed at relieving compression of neural structures and restoring normal CSF dynamics.

Conclusion:

Chiari malformation is characterized by compression of neural structures within the posterior cranial fossa, leading to a variety of neurological symptoms and complications. The compression effects on the brainstem, cranial nerves, cerebellum, and spinal cord can result in deficits in motor coordination, sensory function, and autonomic regulation. Understanding the underlying mechanisms and clinical manifestations of compression effects in Chiari malformation is essential for guiding diagnostic evaluation and therapeutic interventions aimed at improving patient outcomes. Further research into the pathophysiology of compression effects and the development of targeted therapies holds promise for advancing our understanding and management of this complex neurological condition.

Molecular and Cellular Pathways Involved in Chiari Malformation

Chiari malformation is a complex neurological disorder characterized by the downward displacement of the cerebellar tonsils through the foramen magnum, resulting in compression of neural structures and disruption of normal cerebrospinal fluid (CSF) dynamics. While the precise molecular and cellular mechanisms underlying Chiari malformation remain incompletely understood, emerging evidence suggests the involvement of multiple pathways related to craniofacial development, extracellular matrix remodeling, neuronal migration, and neuroinflammation. In this section, we explore the molecular and cellular pathways implicated in the pathogenesis of Chiari malformation, shedding light on the underlying biological processes and potential therapeutic targets.

Craniofacial Developmental Pathways:

The development of the posterior cranial fossa and associated structures is governed by a complex interplay of signaling pathways and transcription factors involved in craniofacial development. Disruptions in these developmental pathways during embryogenesis can lead to abnormalities in the size, shape, and orientation of the posterior cranial fossa, predisposing individuals to Chiari malformation. Several genes implicated in craniofacial development, including PAX1, ZIC1, and TBX1, have been identified as candidate genes for Chiari malformation through genome-wide association studies and genetic linkage analyses. These genes play critical roles in regulating the formation of the cranial base, cranial vault, and associated skeletal structures, highlighting their importance in the pathogenesis of Chiari malformation.

Extracellular Matrix Remodeling:

The extracellular matrix (ECM) is a complex network of proteins and glycosaminoglycans that provides structural support and regulates cellular behavior within tissues. Alterations in ECM composition and remodeling have been implicated in the pathogenesis of Chiari malformation, particularly in the development of craniovertebral abnormalities and alterations in tissue compliance. Abnormalities in genes encoding ECM proteins, such as collagens, elastins, and proteoglycans, have been identified in individuals with Chiari malformation, suggesting a potential role for ECM dysregulation in the pathogenesis of this condition. Additionally, dysregulation of matrix metalloproteinases (MMPs), enzymes involved in ECM remodeling, has been observed in Chiari malformation, further implicating ECM dynamics in the development of this disorder.

Neuronal Migration and Organization:

During embryonic development, neurons within the central nervous system undergo a complex process of migration, differentiation, and organization to form functional neural circuits. Disruptions in neuronal migration and organization have been implicated in the pathogenesis of Chiari malformation, particularly in the development of hindbrain anomalies and cerebellar malformations. Mutations in genes involved in neuronal migration, such as *DCX* (doublecortin) and *REELIN*, have been identified in individuals with Chiari malformation, suggesting a potential role for impaired neuronal migration in the pathogenesis of this condition. Additionally, abnormalities in the development of Purkinje cells, the principal neurons of the cerebellum, have been observed in Chiari malformation, further implicating disruptions in neuronal organization in the pathogenesis of this disorder.

Neuroinflammation and Immune Dysregulation:

Emerging evidence suggests that neuroinflammation and immune dysregulation may contribute to the pathogenesis of Chiari malformation through the activation of inflammatory pathways and the release of pro-inflammatory cytokines. Abnormalities in immune cell infiltration, microglial activation, and cytokine production have been observed in individuals with Chiari malformation, suggesting a potential role for neuroinflammatory processes in the development of this condition. Additionally, genetic variants in immune-related genes, such as *HLA-DQB1* and *TNF*, have been associated with an increased risk of Chiari malformation, further implicating immune dysregulation in the pathogenesis of this disorder.

Therapeutic Implications:

Understanding the molecular and cellular pathways involved in Chiari malformation is essential for identifying potential therapeutic targets and developing targeted interventions to treat this condition. Therapeutic strategies aimed at modulating craniofacial development, ECM remodeling, neuronal migration, and neuroinflammation hold promise for alleviating symptoms and improving outcomes in individuals affected by Chiari malformation. Additionally, advances in genetic screening and personalized medicine may enable the identification of individuals at increased risk of Chiari malformation and the development of tailored therapeutic approaches based on their underlying molecular and cellular pathology.

Conclusion:

Chiari malformation is a complex neurological disorder characterized by the downward displacement of the cerebellar tonsils and compression of neural structures within the posterior cranial fossa. Emerging evidence suggests the involvement of multiple molecular and cellular pathways in the pathogenesis of Chiari malformation, including craniofacial developmental pathways, ECM remodeling, neuronal migration, and neuroinflammation. Understanding the underlying biological processes and molecular mechanisms driving Chiari malformation is essential for developing targeted therapeutic interventions and improving outcomes in individuals affected by this condition. Further research into the molecular and cellular pathways involved in Chiari malformation holds promise for advancing our understanding of this disorder and developing novel therapeutic strategies to address its underlying causes.

CHAPTER 4: CLINICAL PRESENTATION AND DIAGNOSIS

Symptoms and Signs of Chiari Malformation

Chiari malformation is a neurological disorder characterized by the downward displacement of the cerebellar tonsils through the foramen magnum, leading to compression of neural structures within the posterior cranial fossa. This compression can result in a wide range of symptoms and signs, varying in severity and presentation among affected individuals. In this section, we explore the common symptoms and signs associated with Chiari malformation, including neurological deficits, cranial nerve dysfunction, and spinal cord abnormalities, highlighting the clinical manifestations that may prompt diagnostic evaluation and therapeutic intervention.

Headache:

Headache is one of the most common and debilitating symptoms experienced by individuals with Chiari malformation. The headache associated with Chiari malformation is typically described as a persistent, dull, aching pain located at the base of the skull or in the occipital region. The headache may be exacerbated by changes in posture, such as bending forward or straining, and may be accompanied by neck pain or stiffness. The exact mechanism underlying headache in Chiari malformation is not fully understood but is thought to involve compression of neural structures, alterations in cerebrospinal fluid dynamics, and irritation of pain-sensitive structures within the posterior cranial fossa.

Neck Pain and Stiffness:

Neck pain and stiffness are commonly reported symptoms in individuals with Chiari malformation, often accompanying headache and exacerbating discomfort. The neck pain associated with Chiari malformation is typically localized to the cervical spine and may be aggravated by movement or prolonged sitting or standing. Neck stiffness may result from muscle tension, ligamentous strain, or compression of cervical nerve roots by herniated cerebellar tonsils or bony abnormalities within the craniovertebral junction.

Cranial Nerve Dysfunction:

Compression of cranial nerves within the posterior cranial fossa can lead to dysfunction of various cranial nerve functions, resulting in a constellation of symptoms and signs. Cranial nerve dysfunction in Chiari malformation may manifest as:

1. **Dysphagia:** Difficulty swallowing (dysphagia) is a common symptom of Chiari malformation, particularly when compression affects the glossopharyngeal nerve (CN IX), vagus nerve (CN X), or accessory nerve (CN XI). Dysphagia may present as difficulty initiating swallowing, choking or gagging with swallowing, or regurgitation of food or liquids.
2. **Dysarthria:** Impaired speech articulation (dysarthria) may occur in individuals with Chiari malformation due to compression of cranial nerves involved in speech production, such as the hypoglossal nerve (CN XII).

Dysarthria may present as slurred speech, difficulty pronouncing words, or changes in voice quality.
3. **Hoarseness:** Compression of the recurrent laryngeal nerve, a branch of the vagus nerve (CN X), can lead to changes in vocal cord function and hoarseness of voice. Hoarseness may be accompanied by difficulty projecting the voice, reduced vocal range, or vocal fatigue.
4. **Facial Pain or Numbness:** Compression of the trigeminal nerve (CN V) can lead to facial pain, numbness, or sensory disturbances. Facial pain associated with Chiari malformation may be unilateral or bilateral and may involve the distribution of one or more branches of the trigeminal nerve, such as the ophthalmic (V1), maxillary (V2), or mandibular (V3) divisions.

Motor and Sensory Deficits:

Compression of neural structures within the posterior cranial fossa can lead to motor and sensory deficits affecting the upper and lower extremities. Motor deficits may present as weakness, clumsiness, or difficulty with fine motor tasks, particularly in the hands and fingers. Sensory deficits may manifest as numbness, tingling, or loss of sensation in the arms, hands, legs, or feet. The distribution of motor and sensory deficits in Chiari malformation may vary depending on the extent and location of neural compression and may worsen over time if left untreated.

Syringomyelia and Spinal Cord Abnormalities:

Chiari malformation is commonly associated with the development of syringomyelia, a condition characterized by the formation of fluid-filled cavities (syrinxes) within the spinal cord. Syringomyelia may cause additional symptoms and signs, including progressive weakness, sensory loss, or pain in the arms, legs, or trunk. Other spinal cord abnormalities, such as scoliosis or tethered cord syndrome, may also occur in individuals with Chiari malformation and may contribute to neurological deficits and functional impairment.

Autonomic Dysfunction:

Compression of neural structures within the posterior cranial fossa can lead to dysfunction of the autonomic nervous system, resulting in a variety of symptoms affecting cardiovascular, respiratory, gastrointestinal, and genitourinary function. Autonomic dysfunction in Chiari malformation may manifest as dizziness, lightheadedness, palpitations, chest pain, shortness of breath, nausea, vomiting, constipation, urinary retention, or erectile dysfunction. These symptoms may be transient or persistent and may worsen with changes in posture or activity level.

In conclusion, Chiari malformation is associated with a diverse array of symptoms and signs, reflecting the complex neuroanatomical and physiological changes occurring within the posterior cranial fossa. Recognition of the characteristic clinical manifestations of Chiari malformation is essential for prompt diagnosis and appropriate management of affected individuals. Further research into the pathophysiology of Chiari malformation-related symptoms and the development of targeted therapeutic interventions hold promise for improving outcomes and quality of life in individuals affected by this challenging neurological condition.

Diagnostic Imaging Modalities for Chiari Malformation

Chiari malformation is a complex neurological disorder characterized by the downward displacement of the cerebellar tonsils through the foramen magnum, leading to compression of neural structures within the posterior cranial fossa. Accurate diagnosis of Chiari malformation relies on a combination of clinical evaluation and diagnostic imaging modalities that provide detailed anatomical information and allow for the assessment of cerebellar herniation, craniovertebral abnormalities, and associated complications such as syringomyelia. In this section, we explore the diagnostic imaging modalities commonly used in the evaluation of Chiari malformation, highlighting their respective strengths, limitations, and clinical applications.

Magnetic Resonance Imaging (MRI):

Magnetic resonance imaging (MRI) is the gold standard imaging modality for the diagnosis and evaluation of Chiari malformation due to its superior soft tissue contrast and multiplanar imaging capabilities. MRI allows for the visualization of the brain, spinal cord, craniovertebral junction, and associated structures with high spatial resolution, enabling the detection of cerebellar herniation, syringomyelia, and other associated abnormalities. T1-weighted, T2-weighted, and fluid-attenuated inversion recovery (FLAIR) sequences are typically acquired to assess tissue morphology, signal intensity, and CSF flow dynamics. Additionally, advanced MRI techniques such as phase-contrast imaging and cine MRI can be used to evaluate CSF flow dynamics and identify areas of obstruction or flow disturbances within the craniospinal axis.

Computed Tomography (CT) Imaging:

Computed tomography (CT) imaging may be used as an adjunct to MRI in the evaluation of Chiari malformation, particularly in cases where MRI is contraindicated or unavailable. CT imaging provides excellent visualization of bony structures within the craniovertebral junction, allowing for the assessment of basilar invagination, atlantoaxial instability, and other skeletal abnormalities that may predispose to Chiari malformation. Additionally, CT myelography, a specialized imaging technique involving the injection of contrast material into the subarachnoid space, can be used to evaluate CSF flow dynamics and identify areas of obstruction or compression within the spinal canal.

Cine MRI and Phase-Contrast Imaging:

Cine MRI and phase-contrast imaging are specialized MRI techniques used to assess CSF flow dynamics within the craniospinal axis. Cine MRI involves the acquisition of sequential MRI images over time, allowing for the visualization of CSF movement and flow patterns within the subarachnoid space and spinal canal. Phase-contrast imaging utilizes phase shifts in the MRI signal to quantify CSF velocity and flow rates, providing valuable information about CSF dynamics and identifying areas of flow obstruction or turbulence. These advanced imaging techniques are particularly useful for evaluating CSF flow dynamics in individuals with Chiari malformation and may help guide treatment decisions.

Dynamic Imaging Studies:

Dynamic imaging studies, such as upright or dynamic MRI, may be performed to assess changes in CSF dynamics and neural structures with changes in posture or position. Upright MRI allows for imaging of the spine and spinal cord in the weight-bearing position, providing valuable information about the effects of gravity on CSF flow and neural compression. Dynamic MRI studies can help identify positional changes in cerebellar tonsillar descent, spinal cord displacement, or CSF flow obstruction that may not be apparent on conventional supine MRI scans. These dynamic imaging techniques are particularly useful for evaluating symptomatic individuals with positional exacerbation of symptoms or suspected CSF flow abnormalities.

Radiographic Measurements:

Several radiographic measurements may be performed to assess the morphology and dimensions of the posterior cranial fossa and craniovertebral junction. These measurements include the clivoaxial angle, the McRae line, the Boogaard's angle, and the ponticulus posterior. Abnormalities in these measurements, such as a steep clivoaxial angle or a low-lying cerebellar tonsils below the McRae line, may indicate craniovertebral abnormalities or predisposition to Chiari malformation. Radiographic measurements are typically performed on plain radiographs, CT scans, or MRI images and can help guide treatment decisions and surgical planning in individuals with Chiari malformation.

Conclusion:

Diagnostic imaging modalities play a crucial role in the evaluation and diagnosis of Chiari malformation, providing detailed anatomical information and facilitating the assessment of cerebellar herniation, craniovertebral abnormalities, and associated complications. Magnetic resonance imaging (MRI) is the gold standard imaging modality for the diagnosis of Chiari malformation, offering superior soft tissue contrast and multiplanar imaging capabilities. Computed tomography (CT) imaging may be used as an adjunct to MRI for the assessment of bony structures within the craniovertebral junction. Advanced imaging techniques such as cine MRI, phase-contrast imaging, and dynamic imaging studies provide valuable information about CSF flow dynamics and positional changes in neural structures. Radiographic measurements can help identify abnormalities in the posterior cranial fossa and guide treatment decisions in individuals with Chiari malformation. Overall, a multidisciplinary approach involving clinical evaluation and diagnostic imaging is essential for accurate diagnosis and management of Chiari malformation.

Differential Diagnosis of Chiari Malformation

Chiari malformation presents with a constellation of symptoms and signs that overlap with several other neurological, orthopedic, and systemic conditions. As such, accurate diagnosis requires careful consideration of the differential diagnosis to distinguish Chiari malformation from other disorders that may manifest with similar clinical presentations. In this section, we explore the key differential diagnoses of Chiari malformation, highlighting their distinguishing features and diagnostic considerations.

1. Migraine Headache: Migraine headache is a common neurological disorder characterized by recurrent episodes of moderate to severe headache accompanied by nausea, photophobia, and phonophobia. While headache is a predominant symptom of Chiari malformation, distinguishing features of migraine headache include the presence of prodromal symptoms, aura, and triggers such as stress, hormonal changes, or specific foods. Neuroimaging studies, such as MRI, can help differentiate between Chiari malformation and migraine headache by identifying structural abnormalities in the posterior cranial fossa and cerebellar tonsillar descent characteristic of Chiari malformation.

2. Occipital Neuralgia: Occipital neuralgia is a condition characterized by paroxysmal stabbing or shooting pain in the distribution of the occipital nerves, typically radiating from the base of the skull to the occipital region. While occipital neuralgia shares some clinical features with Chiari malformation, such as occipital headache and neck pain, distinguishing features include localized pain along the course of the occipital nerves and tenderness to palpation over the occipital region. Diagnostic nerve blocks or electromyography (EMG) studies may be performed to confirm the diagnosis of occipital neuralgia and differentiate it from Chiari malformation.

3. Cervical Spondylosis: Cervical spondylosis is a degenerative condition characterized by age-related changes in the cervical spine, including disc degeneration, osteophyte formation, and facet joint arthropathy. Symptoms of cervical spondylosis, such as neck pain, radiculopathy, and myelopathy, may overlap with those of Chiari malformation, particularly in cases where cervical cord compression occurs. However, distinguishing features of cervical spondylosis include focal tenderness over the cervical spine, radicular pain radiating into the upper extremities, and neurological deficits consistent with cervical myelopathy. Diagnostic imaging studies, such as MRI or CT myelography, can help identify structural abnormalities in the cervical spine and differentiate cervical spondylosis from Chiari malformation.

4. Syringomyelia: Syringomyelia is a disorder characterized by the formation of fluid-filled cavities (syrinxes) within the spinal cord, often associated with Chiari malformation. While syringomyelia may coexist with Chiari malformation, it can also occur secondary to other conditions such as spinal cord injury, tumor, or arachnoiditis. Distinguishing features of syringomyelia include progressive weakness, sensory loss, or pain in the upper extremities, often accompanied by dissociated sensory deficits and characteristic patterns of sensory impairment. Neuroimaging studies, such as MRI, are essential for confirming the presence of syrinxes within the spinal cord and identifying associated abnormalities, such as Chiari malformation.

5. Basilar Invagination: Basilar invagination is a skeletal abnormality characterized by the upward displacement of the odontoid process into the foramen magnum, resulting in compression of neural structures within the posterior cranial fossa. While basilar invagination shares some clinical features with Chiari malformation, such as headache and cranial nerve dysfunction, distinguishing features include atlantoaxial instability, platybasia (flattening of the skull base), and basilar impression on imaging studies. CT imaging of the craniovertebral junction is essential for confirming the diagnosis of basilar invagination and differentiating it from Chiari malformation.

6. Idiopathic Intracranial Hypertension (IIH): Idiopathic intracranial hypertension (IIH), also known as pseudotumor cerebri, is a condition characterized by elevated intracranial pressure without evidence of an underlying structural abnormality or mass lesion. While IIH shares some clinical features with Chiari malformation, such as headache and visual disturbances, distinguishing features include papilledema (optic disc swelling), transient visual obscurations, and pulsatile tinnitus. Lumbar puncture with measurement of opening pressure is essential for confirming the diagnosis of IIH and ruling out other causes of elevated intracranial pressure, such as Chiari malformation.

7. **Arnold-Chiari Malformation Type II:** Arnold-Chiari malformation type II, also known as Chiari II malformation, is a more severe form of Chiari malformation characterized by downward displacement of the cerebellar vermis, brainstem, and fourth ventricle through the foramen magnum, often associated with myelomeningocele or spina bifida. While Chiari II malformation shares some clinical features with Chiari malformation type I, distinguishing features include the presence of neural tube defects, hydrocephalus, and brainstem abnormalities on imaging studies. MRI of the brain and spine is essential for confirming the diagnosis of Chiari II malformation and identifying associated anomalies.

Conclusion: Accurate diagnosis of Chiari malformation requires careful consideration of the differential diagnosis to differentiate it from other neurological, orthopedic, and systemic conditions that may present with similar symptoms and signs. Key differential diagnoses of Chiari malformation include migraine headache, occipital neuralgia, cervical spondylosis, syringomyelia, basilar invagination, idiopathic intracranial hypertension, and Arnold-Chiari malformation type II. Clinical evaluation, neuroimaging studies, and ancillary diagnostic tests are essential for establishing the correct diagnosis and guiding appropriate management strategies in individuals with suspected

Chiari malformation.

Assessment of Severity and Classification Systems in Chiari Malformation

Chiari malformation is a complex neurological disorder characterized by the downward displacement of the cerebellar tonsils through the foramen magnum, leading to compression of neural structures within the posterior cranial fossa. The severity of Chiari malformation can vary widely among affected individuals, ranging from asymptomatic incidental findings to debilitating neurological deficits and associated complications such as syringomyelia or hydrocephalus. In order to better understand and manage Chiari malformation, various classification systems and severity assessment tools have been developed to categorize the condition based on anatomical features, clinical manifestations, and radiographic findings. In this section, we explore the assessment of severity and classification systems used in Chiari malformation, highlighting their utility in clinical practice and research.

Assessment of Severity:

Assessing the severity of Chiari malformation requires a comprehensive evaluation of clinical symptoms, neurological deficits, radiographic findings, and associated complications. Several factors may influence the severity of Chiari malformation, including the degree of cerebellar herniation, the presence of associated anomalies such as syringomyelia or hydrocephalus, and the presence of neurological symptoms or functional impairment. The severity of Chiari malformation may be categorized as follows:

1. **Asymptomatic Chiari Malformation:** Some individuals with Chiari malformation may remain asymptomatic

throughout their lives and may only be diagnosed incidentally on neuroimaging studies performed for unrelated reasons. Asymptomatic Chiari malformation is typically characterized by mild cerebellar tonsillar descent without associated neurological deficits or clinical symptoms.

2. **Symptomatic Chiari Malformation:** Symptomatic Chiari malformation refers to cases where individuals experience neurological symptoms or functional impairment attributable to the downward displacement of the cerebellar tonsils. Symptoms may include headache, neck pain, cranial nerve dysfunction, motor weakness, sensory deficits, or autonomic dysfunction, and may vary in severity depending on the degree of neural compression and associated complications.

3. **Complicated Chiari Malformation:** Complicated Chiari malformation refers to cases where individuals experience associated complications such as syringomyelia, hydrocephalus, or brainstem compression. Complicated Chiari malformation may present with progressive neurological deficits, worsening symptoms, or functional impairment requiring surgical intervention or specialized management.

Classification Systems:

Several classification systems have been proposed to categorize Chiari malformation based on anatomical features, clinical manifestations, and radiographic findings. These classification systems aim to standardize terminology, facilitate communication among healthcare providers, and guide treatment decisions based on the severity and subtype of Chiari malformation. Some commonly used classification systems in Chiari malformation include:

1. **Chiari Malformation Type I, II, III, and IV:** The

classification system proposed by Hans Chiari in 1891 categorizes Chiari malformation into four types based on the extent of cerebellar herniation and associated anomalies. Chiari malformation type I involves downward displacement of the cerebellar tonsils through the foramen magnum, while type II is characterized by more severe herniation of the cerebellum, brainstem, and fourth ventricle, often associated with myelomeningocele or spina bifida. Chiari malformation type III involves herniation of cerebellar and brainstem tissue into a meningocele or encephalocele, while type IV is characterized by cerebellar hypoplasia or aplasia.

2. **Syringomyelia-Associated Chiari Malformation Classification:** The syringomyelia-associated Chiari malformation classification system proposed by Oldfield and Muraszko categorizes Chiari malformation based on the presence and extent of associated syringomyelia. Type I involves simple descent of the cerebellar tonsils below the foramen magnum without syringomyelia, while type II involves descent of the tonsils with associated syringomyelia extending into the cervical spinal cord. Type III involves descent of the tonsils with a large syrinx extending into the thoracic spinal cord, while type IV involves descent of the tonsils with extensive syringomyelia affecting the entire spinal cord.

3. **Chamberlain's Line and McRae Line Classification:** Chamberlain's line and McRae line are radiographic measurements used to assess the severity of basilar invagination and craniovertebral junction abnormalities in Chiari malformation. Chamberlain's line measures the distance between the opisthion (posterior margin of the foramen magnum) and the basion (anterior margin of the foramen magnum), while McRae line measures the distance between the basion and the posterior-inferior margin of the occiput. Abnormalities in these

measurements may indicate basilar invagination or craniovertebral junction anomalies associated with Chiari malformation.

Clinical Implications:

The assessment of severity and classification of Chiari malformation play a crucial role in guiding treatment decisions, prognostication, and patient counseling. Individuals with asymptomatic Chiari malformation may require periodic clinical and radiographic follow-up to monitor for symptom progression or associated complications. Symptomatic Chiari malformation may be managed conservatively with observation, lifestyle modifications, or symptomatic treatment, while complicated Chiari malformation may require surgical intervention or specialized management to alleviate symptoms, decompress neural structures, and address associated complications such as syringomyelia or hydrocephalus.

Conclusion:

Assessment of severity and classification systems play a vital role in the evaluation and management of Chiari malformation, providing valuable information about anatomical features, clinical manifestations, and associated complications. Clinicians should be familiar with the various classification systems and severity assessment tools used in Chiari malformation to facilitate accurate diagnosis, treatment planning, and patient counseling. Further research and validation of classification systems are needed to improve our understanding of Chiari malformation subtypes and their clinical implications, ultimately leading to better outcomes and quality of life for individuals affected by this challenging neurological condition.

CHAPTER 5: MANAGEMENT STRATEGIES

Conservative Management Approaches for Chiari Malformation

Chiari malformation is a neurological disorder characterized by the downward displacement of the cerebellar tonsils through the foramen magnum, leading to compression of neural structures within the posterior cranial fossa. While surgical intervention may be necessary in cases of symptomatic or complicated Chiari malformation, conservative management approaches play a crucial role in the initial management and long-term care of individuals with Chiari malformation, particularly those with mild symptoms or stable disease. In this section, we explore the various conservative management approaches used in the treatment of Chiari malformation, focusing on lifestyle modifications, pharmacotherapy, and supportive measures aimed at alleviating symptoms and improving quality of life.

Lifestyle Modifications:

Lifestyle modifications are an essential component of conservative management for Chiari malformation, aimed at reducing symptom exacerbation and improving overall well-being. Some key lifestyle modifications for individuals with Chiari malformation include:

1. **Postural Optimization:** Maintaining proper posture and avoiding activities that exacerbate symptoms, such as prolonged sitting, standing, or straining, can help alleviate neck pain, headache, and cranial nerve dysfunction associated with Chiari malformation. Using ergonomic furniture, taking frequent breaks, and practicing relaxation techniques can help reduce musculoskeletal strain and improve comfort.
2. **Weight Management:** Achieving and maintaining a healthy body weight is important for individuals with Chiari malformation, as excess weight can exacerbate symptoms such as headache, neck pain, and fatigue. Adopting a balanced diet, engaging in regular physical activity within the limits of individual tolerance, and seeking guidance from a registered dietitian or nutritionist can help promote weight management and overall health.
3. **Sleep Hygiene:** Ensuring adequate sleep hygiene is essential for individuals with Chiari malformation, as sleep disturbances can exacerbate neurological symptoms and impair cognitive function. Establishing a regular sleep schedule, creating a comfortable sleep environment, and practicing relaxation techniques before bedtime can help improve sleep quality and promote restorative sleep.
4. **Stress Management:** Managing stress and anxiety is important for individuals with Chiari malformation, as psychological stress can exacerbate symptoms and impair coping mechanisms. Engaging in stress-reducing activities such as mindfulness meditation, deep breathing exercises, or psychotherapy can help promote emotional well-being and resilience in the face of chronic illness.

Pharmacotherapy:

Pharmacotherapy may be considered as adjunctive therapy in

the management of specific symptoms associated with Chiari malformation, such as headache, neuropathic pain, or autonomic dysfunction. While pharmacotherapy alone is unlikely to address the underlying structural abnormalities of Chiari malformation, it can help alleviate symptoms and improve quality of life in affected individuals. Some commonly used medications for symptomatic management of Chiari malformation include:

1. **Analgesics:** Nonsteroidal anti-inflammatory drugs (NSAIDs) such as ibuprofen or acetaminophen may be used to relieve headache and neck pain associated with Chiari malformation. Opioid medications may be reserved for severe or refractory pain, but their long-term use should be approached with caution due to the risk of dependence and adverse effects.
2. **Anticonvulsants:** Anticonvulsant medications such as gabapentin or pregabalin may be prescribed for the management of neuropathic pain or sensory disturbances associated with Chiari malformation. These medications work by stabilizing neuronal excitability and reducing abnormal sensory signaling in the central nervous system.
3. **Tricyclic Antidepressants (TCAs):** TCAs such as amitriptyline or nortriptyline may be used to manage neuropathic pain, sleep disturbances, or mood disorders associated with Chiari malformation. TCAs exert analgesic effects through their actions on serotonin and norepinephrine reuptake inhibition, as well as blockade of voltage-gated sodium channels.
4. **Antiemetics:** Antiemetic medications such as ondansetron or prochlorperazine may be prescribed to alleviate nausea and vomiting associated with Chiari malformation, particularly in cases where cranial nerve dysfunction or autonomic dysfunction is present. These medications work by blocking serotonin receptors in the gastrointestinal tract and central nervous system.

Supportive Measures:

In addition to lifestyle modifications and pharmacotherapy, supportive measures are an integral part of conservative management for Chiari malformation, aimed at addressing specific needs and improving overall quality of life. Some supportive measures for individuals with Chiari malformation include:

1. **Physical Therapy:** Physical therapy may be recommended to improve posture, strengthen neck and shoulder muscles, and enhance flexibility and range of motion in individuals with Chiari malformation. Therapeutic exercises, manual therapy techniques, and modalities such as heat or cold therapy can help alleviate musculoskeletal symptoms and improve functional mobility.
2. **Occupational Therapy:** Occupational therapy may be beneficial for individuals with Chiari malformation who experience limitations in activities of daily living due to neurological symptoms or functional impairment. Occupational therapists can provide adaptive equipment, assistive devices, and compensatory strategies to optimize independence and participation in daily activities.
3. **Psychological Support:** Psychological support and counseling may be helpful for individuals with Chiari malformation who experience emotional distress, anxiety, or depression related to their condition. Psychologists, social workers, or mental health counselors can provide coping strategies, stress management techniques, and supportive counseling to address psychosocial needs and promote resilience.
4. **Patient Education:** Patient education is essential for empowering individuals with Chiari malformation to actively participate in their care and make informed decisions about their health. Providing information about

the nature of the condition, expected course of symptoms, available treatment options, and strategies for symptom management can help individuals better understand and cope with their diagnosis.

Conclusion:

Conservative management approaches play a vital role in the initial management and long-term care of individuals with Chiari malformation, particularly those with mild symptoms or stable disease. Lifestyle modifications, pharmacotherapy, and supportive measures are key components of conservative management, aimed at alleviating symptoms, improving quality of life, and optimizing functional outcomes. A multidisciplinary approach involving healthcare providers from various specialties, including neurology, physical therapy, occupational therapy, and psychology, is essential for delivering comprehensive and personalized care to individuals with Chiari malformation. Further research into the efficacy and long-term outcomes of conservative management approaches is needed to optimize treatment strategies and improve outcomes in this patient population.

Surgical Interventions: Indications and Techniques in Chiari Malformation

Chiari malformation is a complex neurological disorder characterized by the downward displacement of the cerebellar tonsils through the foramen magnum, leading to compression of neural structures within the posterior cranial fossa. While conservative management approaches may be effective in alleviating symptoms in some individuals, surgical intervention is often necessary for those with symptomatic or complicated Chiari malformation who fail to respond to conservative measures. In this section, we explore the indications for surgical intervention in Chiari malformation, as well as the various surgical techniques and approaches used to decompress neural structures and alleviate symptoms.

Indications for Surgical Intervention:

Surgical intervention for Chiari malformation is indicated in individuals with symptomatic or complicated disease who experience neurological deficits, severe symptoms, or associated complications such as syringomyelia, hydrocephalus, or brainstem compression. Common indications for surgical intervention in Chiari malformation include:

1. **Symptomatic Chiari Malformation:** Surgical intervention may be indicated in individuals with symptomatic Chiari malformation who experience debilitating neurological symptoms such as severe headache, neck pain, cranial nerve dysfunction, motor weakness, sensory deficits, or autonomic dysfunction that significantly impair quality of life and daily functioning.
2. **Progressive Neurological Deficits:** Surgical intervention may be indicated in individuals with Chiari malformation who experience progressive neurological deficits, worsening symptoms, or functional impairment despite conservative management approaches. Progressive neurological deficits may include worsening motor weakness, sensory loss, or gait disturbances attributable to neural compression or associated complications.
3. **Associated Complications:** Surgical intervention may be indicated in individuals with Chiari malformation who experience associated complications such as syringomyelia, hydrocephalus, or brainstem compression. Surgical decompression of neural structures can help alleviate symptoms, prevent disease progression, and improve long-term outcomes in individuals with

complicated Chiari malformation.

Surgical Techniques and Approaches:

Several surgical techniques and approaches may be employed in the management of Chiari malformation, aimed at decompressing neural structures, restoring normal cerebrospinal fluid dynamics, and alleviating symptoms. The choice of surgical technique depends on individual patient factors, anatomical considerations, and surgeon preference. Some commonly used surgical techniques and approaches for Chiari malformation include:

1. **Posterior Fossa Decompression:** Posterior fossa decompression is the primary surgical intervention for Chiari malformation, aimed at enlarging the posterior cranial fossa to relieve compression of neural structures and restore normal cerebrospinal fluid dynamics. The surgical technique involves removal of a portion of the posterior arch of the atlas (C1) and sometimes the lamina of the axis (C2), as well as the occipital bone and posterior arch of the atlas to create more space for the cerebellum and brainstem. Duraplasty, a procedure in which a patch of dura mater or synthetic material is used to expand the dural sac, may be performed to further enlarge the posterior fossa and prevent cerebrospinal fluid leakage.
2. **Suboccipital Craniectomy:** Suboccipital craniectomy is a surgical technique used to decompress the posterior cranial fossa and create more space for the cerebellum and brainstem. The surgical approach involves removal of a portion of the occipital bone and posterior arch of the atlas (C1) to alleviate compression of neural structures and improve cerebrospinal fluid flow dynamics. Suboccipital craniectomy may be performed alone or in combination with duraplasty to optimize decompression and prevent recurrence of symptoms.

3. **C1 Laminectomy:** C1 laminectomy is a surgical technique used to decompress the neural structures at the craniovertebral junction, particularly in cases of basilar invagination or atlantoaxial instability associated with Chiari malformation. The surgical approach involves removal of the posterior arch of the atlas (C1) to create more space for the cerebellum and brainstem and alleviate compression of neural structures. C1 laminectomy may be performed in combination with posterior fossa decompression or suboccipital craniectomy to achieve optimal decompression and stabilize the craniovertebral junction.

4. **Endoscopic Decompression:** Endoscopic decompression is a minimally invasive surgical technique used to decompress neural structures in Chiari malformation, particularly in cases of limited tonsillar herniation or symptomatic cerebellar ptosis. The surgical approach involves insertion of an endoscope through a small incision in the posterior fossa to visualize and remove obstructing tissue, such as the arachnoid membrane or fibrous bands, and restore normal cerebrospinal fluid flow dynamics. Endoscopic decompression may be performed as a standalone procedure or in combination with other surgical techniques to achieve optimal decompression and symptom relief.

Conclusion:

Surgical intervention plays a crucial role in the management of Chiari malformation, particularly in individuals with symptomatic or complicated disease who fail to respond to conservative measures. Common indications for surgical intervention include symptomatic Chiari malformation, progressive neurological deficits, and associated complications such as syringomyelia or hydrocephalus. Several surgical techniques and approaches may be employed to decompress neural structures, restore normal cerebrospinal fluid dynamics, and alleviate symptoms. The choice of surgical technique depends on individual patient factors, anatomical considerations, and surgeon expertise. Further research and advancements in surgical techniques are needed to optimize outcomes and improve quality of life for individuals with Chiari malformation.

Rehabilitation and Physiotherapy in Chiari Malformation Management

Chiari malformation is a complex neurological disorder characterized by the downward displacement of the cerebellar tonsils through the foramen magnum, leading to compression of neural structures within the posterior cranial fossa. While surgical intervention may be necessary in some cases to alleviate symptoms and prevent disease progression, rehabilitation and physiotherapy play a crucial role in the management of Chiari malformation, particularly in the postoperative period and for individuals with residual symptoms or functional deficits. In this section, we explore the principles and techniques of rehabilitation and physiotherapy in the management of Chiari malformation, focusing on improving functional outcomes, enhancing quality of life, and promoting long-term recovery.

Goals of Rehabilitation and Physiotherapy:

The goals of rehabilitation and physiotherapy in Chiari malformation management are multifaceted, encompassing the following objectives:

1. **Functional Improvement:** Rehabilitation aims to improve functional abilities and enhance independence in activities of daily living for individuals with Chiari malformation. This may include improving mobility, strength, balance, coordination, and proprioception to

facilitate safe and efficient performance of daily tasks.
2. **Symptom Management:** Physiotherapy techniques can help alleviate symptoms such as headache, neck pain, sensory disturbances, and motor weakness associated with Chiari malformation. Therapeutic interventions target specific symptoms and underlying impairments to optimize symptom relief and enhance overall well-being.
3. **Prevention of Complications:** Rehabilitation plays a role in preventing complications such as muscle weakness, joint stiffness, contractures, and secondary musculoskeletal problems that may arise due to immobility or disuse. Physiotherapy interventions aim to maintain joint mobility, prevent muscle atrophy, and optimize musculoskeletal function to minimize the risk of complications.
4. **Optimization of Surgical Outcomes:** Rehabilitation and physiotherapy are integral components of the postoperative management of Chiari malformation, aiming to optimize surgical outcomes, promote healing, and facilitate recovery. Rehabilitation interventions may help reduce postoperative pain, improve surgical wound healing, and restore function following surgery.

Principles of Rehabilitation and Physiotherapy:

Rehabilitation and physiotherapy interventions for Chiari malformation are guided by the following principles:

1. **Individualized Care:** Rehabilitation programs should be tailored to the specific needs, goals, and functional abilities of each individual with Chiari malformation. A comprehensive assessment of impairments, activity limitations, and participation restrictions is essential to develop an individualized treatment plan.
2. **Multidisciplinary Approach:** Rehabilitation of Chiari malformation often involves a multidisciplinary team

of healthcare professionals, including physiotherapists, occupational therapists, speech therapists, psychologists, and social workers. Collaborative care ensures holistic management and addresses the diverse needs of individuals with Chiari malformation.
3. **Evidence-Based Practice:** Rehabilitation interventions should be based on the best available evidence and clinical guidelines to ensure safety, efficacy, and optimal outcomes. Evidence-based practice involves the integration of clinical expertise, patient preferences, and research evidence in decision-making and treatment planning.
4. **Progressive Rehabilitation:** Rehabilitation programs for Chiari malformation typically involve progressive exercise prescription and functional training to gradually increase strength, endurance, and mobility over time. Progressive rehabilitation helps prevent overexertion, minimize risk of injury, and promote long-term adherence to exercise programs.

Rehabilitation Techniques and Interventions:

Rehabilitation and physiotherapy interventions for Chiari malformation may include the following techniques:

1. **Exercise Therapy:** Exercise therapy is a cornerstone of rehabilitation for Chiari malformation, aimed at improving strength, flexibility, endurance, and balance. Therapeutic exercises may include aerobic conditioning, resistance training, stretching, proprioceptive exercises, and balance training to address specific impairments and functional limitations.
2. **Manual Therapy:** Manual therapy techniques such as soft tissue mobilization, joint mobilization, and manual stretching may be used to alleviate muscle tension, improve joint mobility, and reduce pain associated with

Chiari malformation. Manual therapy interventions aim to restore normal musculoskeletal function and optimize movement patterns.

3. **Postural Education and Training:** Postural education and training are essential components of rehabilitation for Chiari malformation, focusing on promoting optimal alignment, posture, and body mechanics to minimize strain on the spine, neck, and shoulders. Ergonomic principles and postural awareness exercises may be incorporated into daily activities to prevent exacerbation of symptoms.

4. **Gait Training:** Gait training is important for individuals with Chiari malformation who experience gait disturbances, imbalance, or coordination deficits. Gait training interventions aim to improve walking patterns, enhance balance control, and reduce fall risk through progressive gait exercises, balance training, and functional mobility tasks.

5. **Pain Management Techniques:** Pain management techniques such as heat therapy, cold therapy, transcutaneous electrical nerve stimulation (TENS), and acupuncture may be used to alleviate headache, neck pain, and musculoskeletal discomfort associated with Chiari malformation. Pain management interventions aim to reduce pain intensity, improve functional mobility, and enhance quality of life.

Conclusion:

Rehabilitation and physiotherapy play a crucial role in the management of Chiari malformation, aiming to improve functional outcomes, alleviate symptoms, and promote long-term recovery. Rehabilitation interventions are individualized, evidence-based, and multidisciplinary, addressing specific impairments, activity limitations, and participation restrictions in individuals with Chiari malformation. Progressive exercise therapy, manual therapy, postural education, gait training, and pain management techniques are key components of rehabilitation programs for Chiari malformation, aiming to optimize functional abilities, enhance quality of life, and promote holistic well-being. A comprehensive, multidisciplinary approach involving collaboration among healthcare professionals and active participation of individuals with Chiari malformation is essential for achieving optimal outcomes and maximizing rehabilitation potential.

Alternative and Complementary Therapies in the Management of Chiari Malformation

Chiari malformation, characterized by the downward displacement of the cerebellar tonsils through the foramen magnum, poses significant challenges in terms of symptom management and quality of life. While surgical intervention and conservative treatments play pivotal roles, many individuals explore alternative and complementary therapies to alleviate symptoms and enhance overall well-being. In this section, we delve into various alternative and complementary therapies used in the management of Chiari malformation, their potential benefits, and their role alongside conventional treatments.

Understanding Alternative and Complementary Therapies:

Alternative and complementary therapies encompass a diverse range of interventions that lie outside the realm of conventional medicine. These therapies may include practices rooted in traditional systems of medicine, mind-body interventions, nutritional approaches, and manual therapies. While some alternative therapies lack scientific evidence of efficacy, others have gained recognition for their potential benefits in symptom management, stress reduction, and holistic well-being.

Common Alternative and Complementary Therapies:

1. **Acupuncture:** Acupuncture, originating from traditional Chinese medicine, involves the insertion of thin needles into specific points on the body to stimulate energy flow and promote healing. Some individuals with Chiari malformation may find acupuncture beneficial for alleviating headache, neck pain, and muscle tension associated with the condition.
2. **Chiropractic Care:** Chiropractic care focuses on the diagnosis and treatment of musculoskeletal disorders through manual manipulation of the spine and joints. While evidence regarding the efficacy of chiropractic care in Chiari malformation is limited, some individuals may seek chiropractic adjustments to alleviate neck pain and improve spinal alignment.
3. **Massage Therapy:** Massage therapy involves manual manipulation of soft tissues to promote relaxation, relieve muscle tension, and improve circulation. Individuals with Chiari malformation may benefit from massage therapy as a complementary approach to alleviate headache, neck pain, and musculoskeletal discomfort.
4. **Yoga and Meditation:** Yoga and meditation practices encompass various mind-body techniques, including postures, breathing exercises, and mindfulness meditation, aimed at promoting physical, mental, and emotional well-being. Some individuals with Chiari malformation may find yoga and meditation beneficial for reducing stress, enhancing relaxation, and improving overall quality of life.
5. **Nutritional Supplements:** Nutritional supplements, such as vitamins, minerals, and herbal remedies, are commonly used as adjunctive therapies in the management of Chiari malformation. While evidence regarding the efficacy of nutritional supplements in Chiari malformation is limited,

some individuals may explore supplements such as magnesium, vitamin B12, or herbal remedies for symptom relief.
6. **Biofeedback Therapy:** Biofeedback therapy involves the use of electronic monitoring devices to provide real-time feedback on physiological parameters such as heart rate, muscle tension, and skin temperature. Individuals with Chiari malformation may use biofeedback therapy to learn self-regulation techniques and reduce symptoms such as headache and stress.

Potential Benefits of Alternative and Complementary Therapies:

While the scientific evidence supporting the efficacy of alternative and complementary therapies in Chiari malformation is limited, some individuals may experience subjective benefits such as:

1. **Symptom Relief:** Certain alternative therapies, such as acupuncture, massage therapy, and chiropractic care, may provide temporary relief from symptoms such as headache, neck pain, and muscle tension, improving overall comfort and well-being.
2. **Stress Reduction:** Mind-body interventions such as yoga, meditation, and biofeedback therapy can help reduce stress, anxiety, and psychological distress associated with chronic illness, promoting relaxation and enhancing coping mechanisms.
3. **Holistic Well-Being:** Alternative and complementary therapies emphasize a holistic approach to health and well-being, addressing physical, mental, and emotional aspects of health. These therapies may empower individuals with Chiari malformation to take an active role in their care and promote self-care practices.
4. **Adjunctive Support:** Alternative and complementary

therapies can complement conventional treatments for Chiari malformation, providing additional support in symptom management, rehabilitation, and overall quality of life enhancement.

Considerations and Precautions:

While alternative and complementary therapies may offer potential benefits, it is essential for individuals with Chiari malformation to exercise caution and consult with healthcare providers before initiating any new treatment modalities. Considerations and precautions include:

1. **Safety:** Some alternative therapies, such as chiropractic manipulation, may pose risks of adverse effects or exacerbation of symptoms in individuals with Chiari malformation. It is important to choose practitioners who are knowledgeable about the condition and its associated risks.
2. **Evidence-Based Practice:** While anecdotal reports and personal testimonials may attest to the benefits of certain alternative therapies, evidence regarding their efficacy in Chiari malformation is often limited. Individuals should approach alternative therapies with a critical eye and prioritize evidence-based practices.
3. **Integration with Conventional Care:** Alternative and complementary therapies should be integrated with conventional treatments for Chiari malformation in a coordinated and collaborative manner. Healthcare providers can help individuals navigate the complex landscape of alternative therapies and make informed decisions about their care.
4. **Individualized Approach:** The choice of alternative therapies should be individualized to the specific needs, preferences, and goals of each individual with Chiari malformation. What works for one person may not

necessarily work for another, and it is important to explore various options and tailor interventions accordingly.

Conclusion:

Alternative and complementary therapies offer a diverse array of approaches to symptom management, stress reduction, and holistic well-being in individuals with Chiari malformation. While the evidence supporting their efficacy may be limited, some individuals may find subjective benefits from these therapies, enhancing their overall quality of life and complementing conventional treatments. It is essential for individuals to approach alternative therapies with caution, consult with healthcare providers, and prioritize evidence-based practices in the management of Chiari malformation. Further research is needed to elucidate the safety, efficacy, and long-term outcomes of alternative and complementary therapies in this complex neurological condition.

CHAPTER 6: COMPLICATIONS AND PROGNOSIS

Neurological Complications of Chiari Malformation

Chiari malformation, characterized by the herniation of cerebellar tonsils through the foramen magnum, can lead to a spectrum of neurological complications. These complications arise due to compression of neural structures within the posterior cranial fossa and may result in a wide range of symptoms and functional impairments. Understanding the neurological complications associated with Chiari malformation is crucial for accurate diagnosis, appropriate management, and optimization of patient outcomes. In this section, we explore the various neurological complications of Chiari malformation, their clinical manifestations, and their implications for patient care.

Compression of Neural Structures:

One of the primary mechanisms underlying neurological complications in Chiari malformation is the compression of neural structures within the posterior cranial fossa. The downward displacement of the cerebellar tonsils can lead to compression of the brainstem, spinal cord, cranial nerves, and blood vessels, resulting in a myriad of neurological symptoms and deficits. The degree of compression and the specific structures affected can vary among individuals with Chiari malformation, contributing to the heterogeneity of clinical presentations.

Clinical Manifestations:

The neurological complications of Chiari malformation can manifest in various ways, depending on the structures affected and the severity of compression. Common clinical manifestations of neurological complications in Chiari malformation include:

1. **Headache:** Headache is one of the most common symptoms of Chiari malformation, typically characterized by occipital or suboccipital pain that may worsen with coughing, straining, or sudden movements. The exact mechanism of headache in Chiari malformation is not fully understood but is believed to be related to traction on pain-sensitive structures within the posterior fossa.
2. **Neck Pain:** Neck pain is frequently reported by individuals with Chiari malformation and may be attributed to muscle tension, cervical instability, or irritation of cervical nerve roots. Neck pain may be exacerbated by prolonged sitting, standing, or neck movements and may coexist with headache or radiate to the shoulders and upper back.
3. **Cranial Nerve Dysfunction:** Compression of cranial nerves within the posterior cranial fossa can lead to various cranial nerve deficits, including facial numbness or weakness (trigeminal nerve), dysphagia or dysarthria (glossopharyngeal and vagus nerves), hoarseness or vocal cord paralysis (recurrent laryngeal nerve), and hearing loss or tinnitus (vestibulocochlear nerve).
4. **Motor Weakness:** Compression of the brainstem or spinal cord in Chiari malformation can result in motor weakness, particularly in the upper extremities. Individuals may experience weakness, clumsiness, or difficulty with fine motor tasks, such as writing or buttoning clothes,

due to impaired motor function secondary to neural compression.

5. **Sensory Disturbances:** Sensory disturbances, such as numbness, tingling, or altered sensation, may occur in the upper and lower extremities due to compression of sensory pathways within the spinal cord or brainstem. Sensory deficits may be unilateral or bilateral and may affect specific dermatomes or sensory modalities.

6. **Gait Ataxia:** Gait ataxia, characterized by unsteadiness, imbalance, and difficulty with coordination and walking, may occur in individuals with Chiari malformation due to compression of the cerebellum or brainstem. Gait ataxia may manifest as wide-based gait, irregular step patterns, or difficulty with tandem walking and may worsen with fatigue or distraction.

7. **Autonomic Dysfunction:** Compression of the brainstem or spinal cord in Chiari malformation can lead to autonomic dysfunction, resulting in symptoms such as dizziness, lightheadedness, syncope, orthostatic hypotension, and disturbances in bowel or bladder function. Autonomic dysfunction may contribute to symptoms of fatigue, malaise, and poor quality of life in affected individuals.

Implications for Patient Care:

The neurological complications of Chiari malformation have significant implications for patient care, including diagnosis, treatment planning, and management strategies. Healthcare providers should be vigilant in recognizing the signs and symptoms of neurological complications and conducting a thorough neurological evaluation to assess the extent of neural compression and associated deficits. Diagnostic imaging modalities, such as magnetic resonance imaging (MRI) of the brain and cervical spine, play a crucial role in identifying structural abnormalities and guiding treatment decisions.

Treatment strategies for neurological complications of Chiari malformation may include:

1. **Surgical Intervention:** Surgical decompression of the posterior cranial fossa is often indicated for individuals with symptomatic Chiari malformation and neurological complications refractory to conservative measures. Posterior fossa decompression surgery aims to alleviate neural compression, restore normal cerebrospinal fluid dynamics, and relieve symptoms.
2. **Conservative Management:** Conservative measures, such as lifestyle modifications, pharmacotherapy, physical therapy, and pain management techniques, may be employed to alleviate symptoms and improve quality of life in individuals with mild to moderate neurological complications of Chiari malformation. These measures may be used alone or in conjunction with surgical intervention, depending on the severity and progression of symptoms.
3. **Rehabilitation:** Rehabilitation and physiotherapy play a crucial role in optimizing functional outcomes and promoting recovery in individuals with neurological complications of Chiari malformation. Rehabilitation interventions focus on improving strength, mobility, balance, coordination, and functional independence through targeted exercises and therapeutic modalities.
4. **Multidisciplinary Care:** The management of neurological complications in Chiari malformation often requires a multidisciplinary approach involving collaboration among neurosurgeons, neurologists, physiatrists, physical therapists, occupational therapists, speech therapists, and other healthcare professionals. Multidisciplinary care ensures comprehensive evaluation, individualized treatment planning, and coordinated management of complex neurological deficits.

Conclusion:

Neurological complications are a hallmark feature of Chiari malformation, stemming from compression of neural structures within the posterior cranial fossa. These complications manifest in diverse ways, including headache, neck pain, cranial nerve dysfunction, motor weakness, sensory disturbances, gait ataxia, and autonomic dysfunction. Recognition of neurological complications is essential for timely diagnosis, appropriate treatment planning, and optimization of patient outcomes. A multidisciplinary approach, incorporating surgical intervention, conservative measures, rehabilitation, and coordinated care, is integral to the management of neurological complications in Chiari malformation, aiming to alleviate symptoms, restore function, and enhance quality of life for affected individuals.

Surgical Complications in Chiari Malformation Management

While surgical intervention is often necessary for individuals with symptomatic Chiari malformation, it is not without risks. Surgical procedures aimed at decompressing neural structures within the posterior cranial fossa carry the potential for complications, ranging from minor to severe. Understanding the possible surgical complications associated with Chiari malformation is essential for informed consent, perioperative management, and optimization of patient outcomes. In this section, we explore the various surgical complications encountered in the management of Chiari malformation, their clinical manifestations, and strategies for prevention and management.

Types of Surgical Complications:

Surgical complications in Chiari malformation management can broadly be categorized into several types, including:

1. **Intraoperative Complications:** Intraoperative complications occur during the surgical procedure and may result from technical challenges, anatomical variations, or unforeseen events. Examples of intraoperative complications include dural tears, hemorrhage, cerebrospinal fluid (CSF) leaks, neural injury, and inadvertent injury to surrounding structures.
2. **Postoperative Complications:** Postoperative complications arise in the immediate aftermath of surgery or during the recovery period and may be related to the surgical procedure itself, patient factors, or perioperative care. Postoperative complications can include CSF leaks, wound infections, meningitis, hydrocephalus, pseudomeningocele formation, neurological deterioration, and hardware-related issues (e.g., hardware migration or failure).
3. **Delayed Complications:** Delayed complications may develop days to weeks after surgery and may be related to inadequate decompression, scar tissue formation, persistent CSF flow abnormalities, or progression of underlying pathology. Delayed complications can manifest as recurrent symptoms, worsening neurological deficits, or the development of new complications requiring further intervention.

Clinical Manifestations:

The clinical manifestations of surgical complications in Chiari malformation management vary depending on the type and severity of the complication. Common clinical manifestations of surgical complications may include:

1. **Worsening Symptoms:** Surgical complications may result in worsening or recurrence of preexisting symptoms associated with Chiari malformation, such

as headache, neck pain, cranial nerve dysfunction, motor weakness, sensory disturbances, gait ataxia, or autonomic dysfunction. Worsening symptoms may indicate inadequate decompression, neural injury, or other postoperative complications requiring further evaluation and management.

2. **New Neurological Deficits:** Surgical complications may lead to the development of new neurological deficits not present before surgery, such as new motor weakness, sensory loss, cranial nerve dysfunction, or changes in gait and coordination. New neurological deficits may indicate nerve injury, spinal cord dysfunction, or other surgical complications requiring prompt assessment and intervention.

3. **CSF Leakage:** CSF leakage is a common complication of posterior fossa decompression surgery in Chiari malformation and may manifest as clear fluid drainage from the surgical incision site, headaches, nausea, vomiting, or signs of meningitis. CSF leakage can lead to increased risk of infection, delayed wound healing, and other complications if not promptly addressed with appropriate measures, such as surgical repair or CSF diversion.

4. **Infection:** Surgical site infections, wound infections, or meningitis may occur as complications of Chiari malformation surgery, particularly in cases of dural tears, CSF leaks, or contamination of the surgical field. Infections may present with fever, localized pain, redness, swelling, drainage, or systemic symptoms and require prompt treatment with antibiotics and wound care to prevent complications.

5. **Hydrocephalus:** Hydrocephalus, characterized by the accumulation of CSF within the ventricular system of the brain, may occur as a surgical complication in Chiari malformation management. Hydrocephalus can

lead to increased intracranial pressure, neurological deterioration, and symptoms such as headache, nausea, vomiting, cognitive changes, or papilledema requiring urgent evaluation and management, including CSF diversion procedures.

Prevention and Management Strategies:

Prevention and management strategies for surgical complications in Chiari malformation management include:

1. **Preoperative Evaluation:** Thorough preoperative evaluation, including neuroimaging studies, neurological assessment, and evaluation of comorbidities, is essential for identifying risk factors, anatomical variations, and potential challenges that may predispose to surgical complications. Preoperative optimization of medical conditions and patient preparation can help minimize the risk of complications.
2. **Surgical Technique:** Attention to surgical technique, meticulous dissection, and careful manipulation of tissues are essential for minimizing the risk of intraoperative complications, such as dural tears, neural injury, or hemorrhage. Surgeons should employ gentle tissue handling, appropriate hemostasis, and precise instrumentation to minimize trauma and ensure adequate decompression.
3. **Intraoperative Monitoring:** Intraoperative monitoring techniques, such as neurophysiological monitoring (e.g., somatosensory evoked potentials, motor evoked potentials), can provide real-time feedback on neurological function and help identify potential intraoperative complications, such as neural injury or ischemia. Intraoperative monitoring allows for timely intervention and modification of surgical technique to mitigate the risk of neurological deficits.

4. **Postoperative Care:** Close postoperative monitoring, including neurological assessment, vital sign monitoring, and surveillance for signs of complications, is essential for early detection and management of postoperative complications. Prompt recognition of complications, such as CSF leaks, infections, or neurological deterioration, allows for timely intervention and optimization of patient outcomes.
5. **Multidisciplinary Collaboration:** Multidisciplinary collaboration among neurosurgeons, neurologists, intensivists, infectious disease specialists, and other healthcare professionals is essential for comprehensive perioperative care, management of surgical complications, and optimization of patient outcomes. Multidisciplinary teams can facilitate timely evaluation, decision-making, and implementation of appropriate interventions in complex cases.

Conclusion:

Surgical complications are inherent risks of Chiari malformation management and can have significant implications for patient outcomes. Understanding the types, clinical manifestations, and prevention strategies for surgical complications is essential for healthcare providers involved in the care of individuals with Chiari malformation. Vigilant perioperative monitoring, meticulous surgical technique, and multidisciplinary collaboration are key components of comprehensive surgical management, aimed at minimizing the risk of complications and optimizing patient safety and outcomes. Despite the potential for complications, surgical intervention remains a crucial component of Chiari malformation management for individuals with symptomatic or progressive disease, offering the potential for symptom relief, neurological improvement, and enhanced quality of life.

Long-Term Prognosis and Quality of Life in Chiari Malformation

Chiari malformation is a complex neurological condition characterized by the downward displacement of the cerebellar tonsils through the foramen magnum, leading to compression of neural structures within the posterior cranial fossa. While surgical intervention and conservative management approaches can help alleviate symptoms and improve outcomes in many cases, the long-term prognosis and quality of life for individuals with Chiari malformation can vary widely. In this section, we explore the factors influencing long-term prognosis, the impact on quality of life, and strategies for optimizing outcomes in Chiari malformation management.

Factors Influencing Long-Term Prognosis:

Several factors influence the long-term prognosis of Chiari malformation, including:

1. **Severity of Symptoms:** The severity and persistence of symptoms at the time of diagnosis can significantly impact long-term prognosis. Individuals with severe, debilitating symptoms, such as intractable headaches, neurological deficits, or associated complications like syringomyelia, may have a poorer prognosis compared to those with mild or intermittent symptoms.
2. **Age at Diagnosis:** The age at which Chiari malformation is diagnosed and treated can influence long-term outcomes. Early diagnosis and intervention may lead to better prognosis and improved outcomes, particularly in pediatric patients, as timely treatment can prevent progression of neurological deficits and associated complications.

3. **Presence of Associated Conditions:** The presence of associated conditions, such as syringomyelia, hydrocephalus, tethered cord syndrome, or craniovertebral junction abnormalities, can impact long-term prognosis and complicate management. Individuals with multiple comorbidities may have a more complex clinical course and may require multidisciplinary care to optimize outcomes.

4. **Effectiveness of Treatment:** The effectiveness of treatment, including surgical intervention and conservative management approaches, plays a crucial role in determining long-term prognosis. Individuals who respond well to treatment and experience symptom relief may have a more favorable prognosis compared to those with persistent or recurrent symptoms despite interventions.

5. **Complications and Recurrence:** The occurrence of surgical complications, recurrence of symptoms, or progression of disease over time can influence long-term prognosis in Chiari malformation. Complications such as CSF leaks, wound infections, neurological deficits, or the need for revision surgery may impact functional outcomes and quality of life.

Impact on Quality of Life:

Chiari malformation can have a profound impact on quality of life, affecting physical, psychological, and social well-being. The following factors contribute to the impact of Chiari malformation on quality of life:

1. **Symptom Burden:** The symptoms associated with Chiari malformation, such as headache, neck pain, cranial nerve dysfunction, motor weakness, sensory disturbances, and gait abnormalities, can significantly impair daily functioning and quality of life. Individuals may experience

limitations in activities of daily living, work, school, and social interactions due to the severity and unpredictability of symptoms.
2. **Functional Impairments:** Neurological deficits resulting from Chiari malformation, such as motor weakness, sensory loss, coordination difficulties, and autonomic dysfunction, can lead to functional impairments and disability. Individuals may struggle with mobility, balance, fine motor skills, and self-care tasks, impacting independence and quality of life.
3. **Psychological Distress:** The chronic nature of Chiari malformation and its associated symptoms can contribute to psychological distress, including anxiety, depression, frustration, and feelings of isolation. Coping with chronic pain, uncertainty about the future, and the challenges of navigating healthcare systems can take a toll on mental health and overall well-being.
4. **Social Impact:** Chiari malformation can disrupt social relationships, recreational activities, and participation in community life. Individuals may experience social withdrawal, stigma, or difficulties in maintaining relationships due to their health condition, leading to feelings of loneliness, isolation, and reduced quality of life.
5. **Treatment Side Effects:** The side effects of treatment for Chiari malformation, such as surgical complications, medication side effects, or limitations in physical activity during recovery, can impact quality of life. Balancing the benefits of treatment with potential risks and adverse effects is essential for optimizing outcomes and preserving quality of life.

Strategies for Optimizing Long-Term Outcomes:

Several strategies can help optimize long-term outcomes and enhance quality of life for individuals with Chiari malformation:

1. **Multidisciplinary Care:** Multidisciplinary care involving neurosurgeons, neurologists, physiatrists, physical therapists, occupational therapists, psychologists, and social workers is essential for comprehensive management of Chiari malformation. A coordinated approach ensures holistic assessment, personalized treatment planning, and ongoing support for individuals and their families.
2. **Patient Education:** Providing education and information about Chiari malformation, its symptoms, treatment options, and self-management strategies empowers individuals to actively participate in their care and make informed decisions. Educating patients and families about warning signs, coping strategies, and resources for support can improve adherence to treatment and enhance self-efficacy.
3. **Symptom Management:** Comprehensive symptom management is essential for improving quality of life and functional outcomes in Chiari malformation. Tailored interventions targeting specific symptoms, such as headache, neck pain, sensory disturbances, or gait abnormalities, can help alleviate discomfort, improve function, and enhance overall well-being.
4. **Rehabilitation and Therapy:** Rehabilitation and therapy play a crucial role in optimizing physical function, mobility, and independence in individuals with Chiari malformation. Physical therapy, occupational therapy, speech therapy, and psychological counseling can address functional impairments, facilitate recovery, and promote adaptive coping strategies.
5. **Psychosocial Support:** Providing psychosocial support, counseling, and access to peer support networks can help individuals cope with the emotional and social challenges of living with Chiari malformation. Addressing psychological distress, promoting resilience, and fostering social connections are important aspects of holistic care

and improving quality of life.

Conclusion:

Chiari malformation can have a significant impact on long-term prognosis and quality of life, affecting physical, psychological, and social well-being. Factors such as symptom severity, age at diagnosis, associated conditions, treatment effectiveness, and complications influence long-term outcomes in Chiari malformation management. Optimizing outcomes requires a multidisciplinary approach, tailored interventions, and ongoing support to address the diverse needs of individuals with Chiari malformation and enhance their overall quality of life. By addressing symptom burden, functional impairments, psychological distress, and social impact, healthcare providers can help individuals with Chiari malformation live well and thrive despite the challenges posed by their condition.

CHAPTER 7: RESEARCH ADVANCES AND FUTURE DIRECTIONS

Current Research Trends and Developments in Chiari Malformation

Chiari malformation, characterized by the herniation of cerebellar tonsils through the foramen magnum, remains a challenging neurological condition with significant variability in clinical presentation, management, and outcomes. Ongoing research efforts seek to elucidate the underlying pathophysiology, refine diagnostic criteria, improve treatment strategies, and enhance our understanding of the long-term implications of Chiari malformation. In this section, we explore current research trends and developments in Chiari malformation, highlighting recent advances, emerging technologies, and areas of investigation shaping the landscape of Chiari research.

Genetic and Molecular Insights:

One area of active research in Chiari malformation focuses on genetic and molecular mechanisms underlying the development and progression of the condition. Genome-wide association studies (GWAS) and next-generation sequencing technologies have identified potential genetic variants associated with Chiari malformation, providing insights into its hereditary and familial predisposition. Researchers are investigating the role of genes involved in craniofacial development, connective tissue integrity, and cerebrospinal fluid dynamics in the pathogenesis of Chiari malformation, with the goal of identifying novel therapeutic targets and personalized treatment approaches.

Neuroimaging Advances:

Advancements in neuroimaging techniques have revolutionized the diagnosis and characterization of Chiari malformation, enabling more precise anatomical evaluation and functional assessment. High-resolution magnetic resonance imaging (MRI), diffusion tensor imaging (DTI), and advanced imaging modalities such as cine MRI and phase-contrast MRI provide detailed information about cerebellar tonsillar descent, craniospinal morphology, CSF flow dynamics, and neural tissue integrity. Researchers are leveraging these imaging modalities to better understand the structural and functional alterations associated with Chiari malformation and their correlation with clinical outcomes, treatment response, and disease progression.

Biomechanical Studies:

Biomechanical studies play a crucial role in elucidating the biomechanics of Chiari malformation, including factors contributing to cerebellar tonsillar herniation, spinal cord compression, and alterations in CSF dynamics. Computational modeling, finite element analysis, and biomechanical simulations are used to investigate the effects of craniospinal morphology, intracranial pressure dynamics, tissue properties, and mechanical forces on the pathogenesis and progression of Chiari malformation. These studies provide valuable insights into the biomechanical factors underlying Chiari malformation and inform the development of predictive models, treatment algorithms, and surgical planning strategies.

Surgical Innovations:

Surgical management remains a cornerstone of Chiari malformation treatment, with ongoing efforts to refine surgical techniques, optimize outcomes, and minimize complications. Innovations in surgical approaches, such as minimally invasive procedures, endoscopic-assisted techniques, and image-guided navigation systems, aim to achieve effective decompression while reducing surgical morbidity and recovery time. Researchers are exploring novel surgical adjuncts, such as duraplasty materials, tissue engineering scaffolds, and biocompatible implants, to enhance dural repair, promote tissue regeneration, and prevent postoperative complications.

Clinical Outcomes Research:

Clinical outcomes research plays a critical role in evaluating the efficacy, safety, and long-term impact of treatment modalities for Chiari malformation. Prospective cohort studies, retrospective analyses, and multicenter collaborations assess treatment outcomes, functional status, quality of life, and patient-reported outcomes following surgical intervention, conservative management, or combination therapies. Researchers investigate factors associated with treatment success, predictors of outcomes, and strategies for optimizing patient care, informed by real-world data and patient experiences.

Translational and Regenerative Medicine:

Translational and regenerative medicine approaches hold promise for addressing the underlying pathophysiology of Chiari malformation and developing novel therapeutic interventions. Preclinical studies using animal models of Chiari malformation explore potential pharmacological agents, cell-based therapies, growth factors, and gene editing techniques to modulate neural tissue remodeling, neuroinflammation, and CSF dynamics. Translation of these preclinical findings to clinical trials offers opportunities for targeted interventions, disease modification, and regenerative strategies aimed at improving outcomes in individuals with Chiari malformation.

Patient-Centered Research:

Patient-centered research initiatives aim to incorporate the perspectives, preferences, and priorities of individuals living with Chiari malformation into research design, implementation, and dissemination. Patient advocacy organizations, online support communities, and patient registries facilitate collaboration between researchers, clinicians, and patients, fostering engagement, empowerment, and shared decision-making. Patient-reported outcomes research, qualitative studies, and participatory research methods capture the lived experiences of individuals with Chiari malformation, inform research priorities, and promote patient-centered care.

Conclusion:

Current research trends and developments in Chiari malformation encompass a multidisciplinary approach, integrating genetic, molecular, neuroimaging, biomechanical, surgical, clinical outcomes, translational, regenerative, and patient-centered research strategies. Advances in these areas hold promise for improving our understanding of Chiari malformation pathogenesis, refining diagnostic criteria, optimizing treatment strategies, and enhancing long-term outcomes and quality of life for affected individuals. Collaborative efforts among researchers, clinicians, patients, and advocacy groups are essential for advancing Chiari research, translating scientific discoveries into clinical practice, and ultimately improving the lives of individuals living with Chiari malformation.

Emerging Therapeutic Strategies for Chiari Malformation

Chiari malformation presents a complex set of challenges in neurological medicine, often requiring a multidisciplinary approach for effective management. While surgical decompression remains the standard treatment for symptomatic cases, emerging therapeutic strategies are being explored to complement existing interventions, improve outcomes, and address unmet needs in Chiari malformation care. In this section, we delve into the latest research and developments in emerging therapeutic strategies for Chiari malformation, including pharmacological, interventional, regenerative, and neuromodulatory approaches.

1. Pharmacological Interventions:

Pharmacological interventions aim to target underlying pathophysiological mechanisms implicated in Chiari malformation, such as altered cerebrospinal fluid dynamics, neuroinflammation, and neuronal dysfunction. Potential pharmacological targets include:

- **CSF Production and Absorption:** Drugs targeting CSF production (e.g., acetazolamide) or absorption (e.g., carbonic anhydrase inhibitors) may modulate CSF dynamics and reduce intracranial pressure, potentially alleviating symptoms associated with Chiari malformation.
- **Neuroinflammation:** Anti-inflammatory agents (e.g., corticosteroids, nonsteroidal anti-inflammatory drugs) may mitigate neuroinflammatory processes implicated in Chiari malformation pathogenesis, reducing neural tissue edema, inflammation, and associated symptoms.
- **Neuronal Excitability:** Agents that modulate neuronal excitability and neurotransmitter function (e.g., gabapentin, pregabalin) may attenuate pain, sensory disturbances, and other neurological symptoms in Chiari malformation through central nervous system

modulation.

Clinical trials evaluating the efficacy and safety of pharmacological interventions in Chiari malformation are underway, aiming to establish evidence-based treatment approaches and optimize patient care.

2. Interventional Procedures:

Interventional procedures offer minimally invasive alternatives to traditional surgical decompression for selected cases of Chiari malformation, particularly those with milder symptoms or contraindications to open surgery. Emerging interventional strategies include:

- **Cervical Epidural Injections:** Cervical epidural steroid injections may provide temporary relief of radicular pain, neck pain, or headache associated with Chiari malformation by reducing inflammation and neural irritation in the cervical spine.
- **Cervical Medial Branch Blocks:** Medial branch blocks targeting the dorsal rami of the cervical spinal nerves may alleviate facet joint-mediated pain in individuals with Chiari malformation, offering symptomatic relief and improving functional outcomes.
- **Nerve Root Decompression:** Percutaneous decompression techniques, such as foraminal nerve root decompression or selective nerve root blocks, may relieve radicular symptoms and neural compression in Chiari malformation by addressing foraminal stenosis or nerve root impingement.

These interventional procedures are typically performed under fluoroscopic guidance or ultrasound visualization, offering a less invasive alternative to surgical decompression for certain patients with Chiari malformation.

3. Regenerative Medicine Approaches:

Regenerative medicine holds promise for addressing structural abnormalities, promoting tissue repair, and restoring normal anatomy and function in Chiari malformation. Emerging regenerative strategies include:

- **Stem Cell Therapy:** Stem cell-based approaches aim to harness the regenerative potential of stem cells to promote tissue regeneration, neuroprotection, and neural tissue remodeling in Chiari malformation. Preclinical studies using stem cell transplantation have shown promising results in animal models, suggesting potential applications for tissue repair and regeneration in humans.
- **Tissue Engineering:** Tissue engineering approaches involve the development of biomimetic scaffolds, bioactive materials, and tissue-engineered constructs to facilitate tissue repair, dural reconstruction, and spinal cord regeneration in Chiari malformation. These innovative strategies offer opportunities for customized treatment approaches and personalized regenerative therapies.

Clinical translation of regenerative medicine approaches for Chiari malformation requires further investigation, including rigorous preclinical studies, optimization of delivery methods, and evaluation of safety and efficacy in clinical trials.

4. Neuromodulation Techniques:

Neuromodulation techniques aim to modulate neural activity, neural pathways, or neurophysiological processes implicated in Chiari malformation to alleviate symptoms and improve functional outcomes. Emerging neuromodulation strategies include:

- **Transcutaneous Electrical Nerve Stimulation (TENS):** TENS therapy delivers low-frequency electrical

stimulation to peripheral nerves or specific dermatomes, modulating pain perception, sensory processing, and neural signaling pathways implicated in Chiari malformation-related symptoms such as headache, neck pain, or neuropathic pain.
- **Spinal Cord Stimulation (SCS):** SCS delivers electrical stimulation to the dorsal columns of the spinal cord, modulating pain transmission and central sensitization processes involved in Chiari malformation-related pain syndromes. SCS may offer symptomatic relief and functional improvement in individuals with refractory pain despite conventional treatments.

These neuromodulation techniques are noninvasive or minimally invasive and may be used as adjunctive therapies to complement existing treatments or as standalone interventions for selected patients with Chiari malformation.

Conclusion:

Emerging therapeutic strategies for Chiari malformation encompass a diverse array of approaches, ranging from pharmacological interventions and interventional procedures to regenerative medicine and neuromodulation techniques. These innovative strategies hold promise for expanding treatment options, improving outcomes, and addressing unmet needs in Chiari malformation management. Clinical translation of emerging therapeutic approaches requires rigorous evaluation in preclinical and clinical studies to establish safety, efficacy, and long-term benefits for individuals living with Chiari malformation. Collaborative efforts among researchers, clinicians, industry partners, and patient advocates are essential for advancing the field and bringing novel therapies to fruition, ultimately improving the lives of individuals affected by Chiari malformation.

Challenges and Opportunities in Chiari Malformation Research

Chiari malformation presents a complex and multifaceted challenge in the field of neurological medicine, characterized by anatomical abnormalities, neurological symptoms, and variable clinical outcomes. While significant progress has been made in understanding the pathophysiology, diagnosis, and management of Chiari malformation, several challenges persist, alongside opportunities for innovation and advancement. In this section, we explore the key challenges and opportunities in Chiari malformation research, highlighting areas of unmet need, emerging trends, and future directions for improving patient care and outcomes.

1. Understanding Pathophysiology:

Challenges: Despite advances in neuroimaging and molecular biology, the precise pathophysiological mechanisms underlying Chiari malformation remain incompletely understood. The interplay between craniospinal morphology, cerebrospinal fluid dynamics, tissue biomechanics, and genetic factors contributing to cerebellar herniation and neural compression is complex and multifactorial.

Opportunities: Emerging technologies, such as advanced neuroimaging techniques, computational modeling, and genomic studies, offer opportunities to unravel the underlying pathophysiology of Chiari malformation. Integrating multidisciplinary approaches, including genetics, biomechanics, and neurophysiology, may provide insights into disease mechanisms and identify novel therapeutic targets.

2. Improving Diagnostic Accuracy:

Challenges: Accurate diagnosis of Chiari malformation relies on comprehensive clinical evaluation and neuroimaging assessment, yet diagnostic criteria and classification systems continue to evolve. Variability in imaging protocols, observer interpretation, and clinical phenotypes pose challenges to standardization and consistency in diagnosis.

Opportunities: Advancements in neuroimaging technology, such as high-resolution MRI, quantitative imaging biomarkers, and machine learning algorithms, offer opportunities to improve diagnostic accuracy and phenotypic characterization of Chiari malformation. Collaborative efforts to develop consensus guidelines, standardized protocols, and diagnostic criteria may enhance diagnostic reliability and facilitate early intervention.

3. Tailoring Treatment Approaches:

Challenges: Treatment decisions in Chiari malformation management are often guided by symptom severity, anatomical characteristics, and patient preferences, yet there is a lack of consensus on optimal treatment algorithms and individualized approaches. Variability in treatment outcomes, complications, and long-term efficacy underscores the need for personalized therapeutic strategies.

Opportunities: Precision medicine approaches, incorporating patient-specific factors, imaging biomarkers, genetic profiles, and functional assessments, hold promise for tailoring treatment approaches to the unique needs of individuals with Chiari malformation. Prospective studies, registries, and clinical trials evaluating stratified treatment strategies may identify predictors of treatment response and optimize therapeutic outcomes.

4. Addressing Comorbidities and Complications:

Challenges: Chiari malformation often coexists with other neurological conditions, such as syringomyelia, hydrocephalus, tethered cord syndrome, and craniovertebral junction abnormalities, complicating management and prognostication. Surgical complications, recurrence of symptoms, and long-term sequelae pose challenges to optimal patient outcomes.

Opportunities: Comprehensive multidisciplinary care, involving neurosurgeons, neurologists, physiatrists, therapists, and allied health professionals, is essential for addressing comorbidities, optimizing perioperative management, and managing complications in Chiari malformation. Integrated care models, collaborative care pathways, and shared decision-making frameworks may improve coordination, communication, and continuity of care for individuals with complex needs.

5. Advancing Research Infrastructure:

Challenges: Limited research funding, fragmented data repositories, and lack of centralized research infrastructure present barriers to collaborative research efforts, data sharing, and dissemination of findings in Chiari malformation research. Small sample sizes, retrospective study designs, and heterogeneity in study populations hinder generalizability and reproducibility of research findings.

Opportunities: Investing in dedicated research funding, establishing multicenter collaborations, and leveraging existing resources, such as patient registries and biobanks, can enhance research infrastructure and facilitate large-scale studies in Chiari malformation. Open-access data repositories, standardized data collection tools, and collaborative platforms promote transparency, reproducibility, and data sharing across research communities.

6. Patient-Centered Research and Advocacy:

Challenges: Limited patient engagement, lack of awareness, and underrepresentation of patient perspectives in research design and prioritization pose challenges to patient-centered care and advocacy efforts in Chiari malformation. Disparities in access to care, socioeconomic factors, and healthcare disparities contribute to inequities in disease management and outcomes.

Opportunities: Empowering individuals with Chiari malformation as partners in research, advocacy, and healthcare decision-making fosters patient-centered approaches, promotes shared decision-making, and enhances patient satisfaction and outcomes. Patient advocacy organizations, support groups, and online communities play a crucial role in raising awareness, promoting education, and amplifying patient voices in Chiari malformation research and healthcare policy.

Conclusion:

Addressing the challenges and opportunities in Chiari malformation research requires a concerted effort from researchers, clinicians, patients, advocates, and policymakers. By advancing our understanding of disease mechanisms, improving diagnostic accuracy, tailoring treatment approaches, addressing comorbidities, enhancing research infrastructure, and promoting patient-centered care, we can make meaningful strides towards improving outcomes and quality of life for individuals living with Chiari malformation. Collaborative multidisciplinary efforts, innovative research methodologies, and advocacy for patient engagement and equity are essential for realizing the full potential of Chiari malformation research and translating scientific discoveries into tangible benefits for those affected by the condition.

CHAPTER 8: HOLISTIC APPROACHES TO CHIARI MALFORMATION MANAGEMENT

Nutritional Considerations in Chiari Malformation

Nutrition plays a crucial role in supporting overall health and well-being, and it is particularly important for individuals living with Chiari malformation. While nutrition alone may not directly treat Chiari malformation, adopting a balanced diet and addressing specific nutritional considerations can help optimize health, manage symptoms, and enhance quality of life. In this section, we explore the nutritional considerations relevant to Chiari malformation, including dietary strategies, hydration, supplementation, and potential interactions with symptom management.

1. Balanced Diet:

A balanced diet rich in essential nutrients is fundamental for supporting overall health and managing symptoms associated with Chiari malformation. Key components of a balanced diet include:

- **Fruits and Vegetables:** Incorporating a variety of fruits and vegetables provides essential vitamins, minerals, antioxidants, and fiber, which support immune function, reduce inflammation, and promote gastrointestinal health.
- **Whole Grains:** Whole grains, such as brown rice, quinoa, oats, and whole wheat, are excellent sources of complex carbohydrates, fiber, and B vitamins, which help maintain energy levels, stabilize blood sugar, and support neurological function.
- **Lean Proteins:** Lean protein sources, such as poultry, fish, tofu, legumes, and nuts, provide essential amino acids necessary for tissue repair, muscle maintenance, and neurotransmitter synthesis.
- **Healthy Fats:** Including sources of healthy fats, such as olive oil, avocado, nuts, seeds, and fatty fish, supports brain health, reduces inflammation, and helps maintain cardiovascular health.
- **Hydration:** Adequate hydration is essential for maintaining optimal hydration status, supporting cerebrospinal fluid dynamics, and preventing dehydration-related symptoms such as headache and fatigue. Drinking plenty of water throughout the day and limiting caffeine and alcohol intake can help ensure adequate hydration.

2. Symptom Management:

Certain dietary factors may influence symptoms commonly associated with Chiari malformation, such as headache, gastrointestinal disturbances, and sleep disturbances. Considerations for symptom management include:

- **Headache Management:** Some individuals with Chiari

malformation may experience headaches triggered by certain foods or additives, such as caffeine, artificial sweeteners, nitrates, and MSG. Keeping a food diary to identify potential triggers and avoiding known triggers may help alleviate headache symptoms.

- **Gastrointestinal Health:** Gastrointestinal symptoms, such as nausea, vomiting, reflux, and constipation, are common in Chiari malformation and may be influenced by dietary factors. Eating smaller, more frequent meals, avoiding spicy or greasy foods, and incorporating fiber-rich foods can help support gastrointestinal health and alleviate symptoms.
- **Sleep Quality:** Diet and nutrition can impact sleep quality and overall sleep hygiene, which may affect symptom severity and quality of life in individuals with Chiari malformation. Avoiding heavy meals, caffeine, and alcohol close to bedtime, and incorporating sleep-promoting foods such as complex carbohydrates, protein, and magnesium-rich foods, can support restful sleep.

3. Supplementation:

In some cases, supplementation with specific nutrients may be beneficial for individuals with Chiari malformation, particularly if dietary intake is inadequate or if certain nutritional deficiencies are identified. Common supplements that may be considered include:

- **Vitamin D:** Vitamin D deficiency is prevalent in the general population and has been associated with various neurological conditions. Supplementing with vitamin D may help support bone health, immune function, and neurological well-being, particularly in individuals with limited sun exposure or malabsorption issues.
- **Omega-3 Fatty Acids:** Omega-3 fatty acids, found in fish oil supplements, have anti-inflammatory properties and

may help reduce inflammation, support cardiovascular health, and promote cognitive function. Supplementing with omega-3 fatty acids may be beneficial for individuals with Chiari malformation, especially those with inflammatory or neurological symptoms.
- **Magnesium:** Magnesium plays a crucial role in muscle function, nerve transmission, and relaxation, and deficiency may contribute to symptoms such as muscle cramps, headaches, and sleep disturbances. Supplementing with magnesium may help alleviate these symptoms and support overall well-being.

4. Individualized Approach:

It is important to emphasize that nutritional needs and dietary preferences vary among individuals, and there is no one-size-fits-all approach to nutrition in Chiari malformation. Consulting with a registered dietitian or nutritionist who specializes in neurological conditions can help develop personalized dietary recommendations tailored to individual needs, preferences, and health goals.

Conclusion:

Nutrition plays a critical role in supporting overall health and well-being in individuals with Chiari malformation. Adopting a balanced diet, addressing specific nutritional considerations, and incorporating symptom management strategies can help optimize health, manage symptoms, and enhance quality of life. While nutrition alone may not cure Chiari malformation, it can complement other treatment modalities and support overall wellness. By taking a holistic approach to nutrition and incorporating evidence-based dietary strategies, individuals with Chiari malformation can take proactive steps to support their health and well-being.

Mind-Body Techniques for Pain Management in Chiari Malformation

Pain management is a significant aspect of Chiari malformation treatment, as individuals with this condition often experience chronic headaches, neck pain, and other types of discomfort. While traditional medical interventions play a crucial role in pain management, mind-body techniques offer complementary approaches that can help alleviate symptoms, improve coping mechanisms, and enhance overall well-being. In this section, we explore various mind-body techniques for pain management in Chiari malformation, including relaxation techniques, mindfulness practices, biofeedback, and cognitive-behavioral strategies.

1. Relaxation Techniques:

Relaxation techniques aim to promote physical and mental relaxation, reduce muscle tension, and alleviate stress, all of which can contribute to pain relief in individuals with Chiari malformation. Common relaxation techniques include:

- **Deep Breathing:** Deep breathing exercises involve slow, deep inhalation through the nose, followed by a gradual exhalation through the mouth. This technique helps activate the body's relaxation response, reduce sympathetic nervous system activity, and promote feelings of calmness and relaxation.
- **Progressive Muscle Relaxation (PMR):** PMR involves systematically tensing and then relaxing different muscle groups throughout the body, typically starting from the toes and progressing to the head. By alternating between muscle tension and relaxation, PMR helps individuals become more aware of muscle tension and release it

effectively.
- **Guided Imagery:** Guided imagery involves visualizing calming and peaceful scenes or experiences, such as a tranquil beach or a serene forest. By engaging the imagination and focusing on positive sensory experiences, guided imagery can help distract from pain, reduce anxiety, and promote relaxation.

2. Mindfulness Practices:

Mindfulness practices cultivate present-moment awareness, nonjudgmental acceptance, and compassionate self-care, which can be particularly beneficial for individuals managing chronic pain associated with Chiari malformation. Key mindfulness practices include:

- **Mindful Meditation:** Mindful meditation involves paying attention to the present moment, including sensations, thoughts, and emotions, without judgment or attachment. By cultivating mindfulness through meditation practice, individuals can develop greater resilience to pain, reduce reactivity to symptoms, and enhance emotional well-being.
- **Body Scan:** Body scan meditation involves systematically scanning through different parts of the body, observing sensations, tensions, and areas of discomfort. By increasing awareness of bodily sensations and promoting relaxation, the body scan technique can help individuals manage pain and improve body awareness.
- **Mindful Movement:** Mindful movement practices, such as yoga, tai chi, or qigong, combine gentle physical movements with mindfulness and breath awareness. These practices promote flexibility, strength, and balance while fostering relaxation, stress reduction, and pain management.

3. Biofeedback:

Biofeedback is a technique that enables individuals to monitor and control physiological processes, such as heart rate, muscle tension, and skin temperature, through real-time feedback provided by electronic monitoring devices. Biofeedback training teaches individuals to recognize and modify physiological responses associated with pain, stress, and tension, leading to improved pain management and self-regulation.

- **Electromyographic (EMG) Biofeedback:** EMG biofeedback measures muscle activity and tension levels, providing visual or auditory feedback to help individuals learn to relax muscles and reduce tension. EMG biofeedback can be particularly beneficial for individuals with Chiari malformation who experience muscle spasms, tension headaches, or neck pain.
- **Temperature Biofeedback:** Temperature biofeedback measures changes in skin temperature, which can reflect levels of peripheral blood flow and relaxation. By learning to increase peripheral blood flow and promote relaxation, individuals can reduce pain perception and improve overall well-being.

4. Cognitive-Behavioral Strategies:

Cognitive-behavioral strategies focus on changing negative thought patterns, beliefs, and behaviors associated with pain, stress, and emotional distress. By addressing cognitive distortions and maladaptive coping strategies, cognitive-behavioral techniques can help individuals with Chiari malformation manage pain more effectively and improve psychological well-being.

- **Cognitive Restructuring:** Cognitive restructuring involves identifying and challenging negative or irrational thoughts related to pain, such as catastrophizing, overgeneralization, or all-or-nothing thinking. By replacing negative thoughts with more balanced and realistic perspectives, individuals can reduce emotional distress and improve pain coping strategies.

- **Pain Coping Skills Training:** Pain coping skills training teaches individuals practical strategies for managing pain, such as relaxation techniques, distraction techniques, pacing activities, and problem-solving skills. By acquiring effective pain coping skills, individuals can regain a sense of control over their symptoms and improve their ability to function despite pain.
- **Activity Pacing:** Activity pacing involves balancing rest and activity to avoid overexertion and exacerbation of symptoms while maintaining functional independence. By pacing activities and taking regular breaks, individuals can conserve energy, reduce pain flare-ups, and maintain a more sustainable level of activity.

Conclusion:

Mind-body techniques offer valuable tools for pain management in individuals with Chiari malformation, complementing traditional medical interventions and promoting holistic well-being. By incorporating relaxation techniques, mindfulness practices, biofeedback, and cognitive-behavioral strategies into their pain management regimen, individuals with Chiari malformation can improve symptom control, enhance coping mechanisms, and foster a greater sense of empowerment and resilience in the face of chronic pain. Working with healthcare providers, therapists, and support networks can help individuals tailor mind-body techniques to their specific needs and preferences, maximizing their effectiveness in managing Chiari-related pain and optimizing overall quality of life.

Lifestyle Modifications and Stress Reduction in Chiari Malformation Management

Living with Chiari malformation presents unique challenges that can impact various aspects of daily life, including physical health, emotional well-being, and overall quality of life. While medical interventions are essential for managing symptoms and addressing structural abnormalities, lifestyle modifications and stress reduction techniques play a crucial role in supporting optimal health, minimizing symptom exacerbation, and promoting holistic well-being. In this section, we explore the importance of lifestyle modifications and stress reduction strategies in Chiari malformation management, focusing on key areas such as physical activity, sleep hygiene, nutrition, stress management, and self-care practices.

1. Physical Activity:

Regular physical activity is essential for maintaining mobility, strength, flexibility, and cardiovascular health, all of which contribute to overall well-being in individuals with Chiari malformation. However, it is important to approach physical activity with caution and adapt activities to individual capabilities and symptom severity. Key considerations for physical activity in Chiari malformation management include:

- **Low-Impact Exercises:** Engaging in low-impact exercises such as walking, swimming, cycling, and gentle yoga can help improve cardiovascular fitness, muscle tone, and joint mobility without placing excessive strain on the spine or exacerbating symptoms.
- **Core Strengthening:** Strengthening the core muscles, including the abdominal and back muscles, can provide stability and support to the spine, reducing the risk of

postural abnormalities and alleviating strain on the neck and upper back.
- **Flexibility and Range of Motion:** Incorporating stretching and range-of-motion exercises into daily routines can help maintain flexibility, prevent muscle stiffness, and reduce the risk of musculoskeletal complications associated with Chiari malformation.

2. Sleep Hygiene:

Quality sleep is essential for overall health and well-being, yet individuals with Chiari malformation may experience sleep disturbances due to pain, discomfort, or neurological symptoms. Adopting good sleep hygiene practices can promote restful sleep and improve sleep quality. Key strategies for optimizing sleep hygiene include:

- **Establishing a Regular Sleep Schedule:** Maintaining a consistent sleep schedule by going to bed and waking up at the same time each day helps regulate the body's internal clock and promotes healthy sleep-wake cycles.
- **Creating a Relaxing Sleep Environment:** Creating a comfortable and conducive sleep environment, with a cool, dark, and quiet bedroom, can help promote relaxation and signal the body that it is time to sleep.
- **Limiting Stimulants Before Bedtime:** Avoiding caffeine, nicotine, and electronic devices with blue light emission close to bedtime can help reduce arousal and promote relaxation before sleep.

3. Nutrition:

A balanced and nutritious diet plays a vital role in supporting overall health, managing symptoms, and promoting recovery in individuals with Chiari malformation. While there is no specific diet that is universally recommended for Chiari malformation, adopting a diet rich in whole foods, fruits, vegetables, lean proteins, and healthy fats can provide essential nutrients and support overall well-being. Key nutritional considerations include:

- **Hydration:** Staying adequately hydrated is important for maintaining optimal cerebrospinal fluid dynamics, preventing dehydration-related symptoms, and supporting overall health. Drinking plenty of water throughout the day is essential, particularly in individuals with Chiari malformation who may be prone to headaches and fatigue.
- **Balanced Macronutrients:** Consuming a balanced ratio of macronutrients, including carbohydrates, proteins, and fats, helps provide sustained energy levels, support muscle function, and regulate metabolism.
- **Anti-Inflammatory Foods:** Incorporating anti-inflammatory foods such as fatty fish, nuts, seeds, fruits, vegetables, and whole grains can help reduce inflammation, support immune function, and alleviate symptoms associated with Chiari malformation.

4. Stress Management:

Chronic pain, neurological symptoms, and functional limitations associated with Chiari malformation can contribute to stress and emotional distress. Effective stress management techniques can help individuals cope with symptoms, reduce anxiety, and improve overall well-being. Key strategies for stress management include:

- **Mindfulness and Relaxation Techniques:** Practicing mindfulness meditation, deep breathing exercises, progressive muscle relaxation, guided imagery, and other relaxation techniques can promote relaxation, reduce muscle tension, and alleviate stress.
- **Cognitive-Behavioral Therapy (CBT):** CBT is a therapeutic

approach that helps individuals identify and challenge negative thought patterns, develop coping skills, and cultivate adaptive responses to stressors. CBT techniques can be particularly beneficial for managing pain, anxiety, and depression in individuals with Chiari malformation.
- **Social Support and Connection:** Building a strong support network of family, friends, healthcare providers, and peer support groups can provide emotional support, practical assistance, and validation of experiences, reducing feelings of isolation and promoting resilience.

5. Self-Care Practices:

Self-care practices are essential for nurturing physical, emotional, and psychological well-being in individuals with Chiari malformation. Engaging in self-care activities that promote relaxation, enjoyment, and self-expression can enhance overall quality of life. Key self-care practices include:

- **Hobbies and Creative Activities:** Engaging in hobbies, creative pursuits, and leisure activities that bring joy, fulfillment, and a sense of accomplishment can help individuals cope with stress, distract from symptoms, and foster a positive outlook on life.
- **Mind-Body Practices:** Incorporating mind-body practices such as yoga, tai chi, qigong, or dance therapy can promote relaxation, body awareness, and emotional expression, enhancing overall well-being and resilience.
- **Nature and Outdoor Activities:** Spending time in nature, enjoying outdoor activities, and connecting with the natural world can provide a sense of peace, rejuvenation, and connection, reducing stress and enhancing mood.

Conclusion:

Lifestyle modifications and stress reduction techniques are integral components of Chiari malformation management, supporting overall health, symptom management, and quality of life. By incorporating physical activity, sleep hygiene, nutrition, stress management, and self-care practices into daily routines, individuals with Chiari malformation can optimize their well-being, improve symptom control, and enhance resilience in the face of chronic illness. Working collaboratively with healthcare providers, therapists, and support networks can help individuals develop personalized strategies for lifestyle modifications and stress reduction, empowering them to take an active role in managing their health and maximizing their quality of life.

Integrative Medicine Approaches in Chiari Malformation Management

Integrative medicine encompasses a holistic approach to healthcare that combines conventional medical treatments with complementary and alternative therapies to address the physical, emotional, and spiritual aspects of health and healing. In the context of Chiari malformation management, integrative medicine offers a diverse array of approaches that aim to complement traditional medical interventions, alleviate symptoms, improve quality of life, and promote overall well-being. In this section, we explore various integrative medicine approaches relevant to Chiari malformation, including acupuncture, chiropractic care, herbal medicine, mind-body practices, and holistic therapies.

1. Acupuncture:

Acupuncture is a traditional Chinese medicine technique that involves the insertion of thin needles into specific points on the body to stimulate energy flow, balance Qi (vital energy), and promote healing. In individuals with Chiari malformation, acupuncture may help alleviate pain, reduce muscle tension, improve circulation, and enhance overall well-being. Research suggests that acupuncture may modulate pain perception, regulate neuroendocrine pathways, and promote relaxation, making it a potentially beneficial adjunctive therapy for pain management in Chiari malformation.

2. Chiropractic Care:

Chiropractic care focuses on the diagnosis, treatment, and prevention of musculoskeletal disorders, with an emphasis on spinal alignment, joint mobilization, and manual therapy techniques. In individuals with Chiari malformation, chiropractic care may help address spinal misalignments, alleviate musculoskeletal symptoms, and improve biomechanical function. While the evidence supporting the effectiveness of chiropractic care in Chiari malformation is limited, some individuals may experience symptom relief and improved functional outcomes with chiropractic adjustments and adjunctive therapies such as soft tissue manipulation, therapeutic exercises, and lifestyle counseling.

3. Herbal Medicine:

Herbal medicine involves the use of plant-based remedies, botanical extracts, and natural substances to promote health, prevent illness, and alleviate symptoms. In Chiari malformation management, herbal medicine may offer potential benefits for symptom management, immune support, and overall well-being. Common herbs and botanicals used in Chiari malformation management include:

- **Turmeric:** Turmeric contains curcumin, a compound with anti-inflammatory and antioxidant properties that may help reduce inflammation, alleviate pain, and support neurological health in individuals with Chiari malformation.
- **Ginger:** Ginger has anti-inflammatory and analgesic

properties that may help alleviate headache, nausea, and gastrointestinal symptoms associated with Chiari malformation.
- **Ginkgo Biloba:** Ginkgo biloba is thought to improve cerebral blood flow, cognitive function, and neurological symptoms in individuals with Chiari malformation, although further research is needed to confirm its efficacy.

4. Mind-Body Practices:

Mind-body practices encompass a diverse range of techniques that integrate the mind and body to promote health, healing, and well-being. In individuals with Chiari malformation, mind-body practices such as meditation, yoga, tai chi, and qigong may help reduce stress, improve pain management, enhance relaxation, and foster emotional resilience. These practices emphasize breath awareness, mindfulness, movement, and body awareness, providing individuals with valuable tools for self-care, stress reduction, and symptom management.

5. Holistic Therapies:

Holistic therapies take a comprehensive approach to health and healing, addressing the physical, emotional, mental, and spiritual aspects of well-being. In Chiari malformation management, holistic therapies such as massage therapy, aromatherapy, Reiki, and energy healing may help promote relaxation, reduce pain, alleviate stress, and enhance overall quality of life. These therapies aim to restore balance, harmony, and vitality to the body, mind, and spirit, supporting individuals on their journey toward healing and wellness.

Conclusion:

Integrative medicine approaches offer valuable tools and techniques for managing Chiari malformation, complementing traditional medical interventions and addressing the diverse needs of individuals living with this condition. By incorporating acupuncture, chiropractic care, herbal medicine, mind-body practices, and holistic therapies into their treatment regimen, individuals with Chiari malformation can access a broad spectrum of resources and support for symptom management, pain relief, and overall well-being. It is essential for individuals to work collaboratively with healthcare providers, integrative medicine practitioners, and other members of their healthcare team to develop personalized treatment plans that integrate conventional and complementary approaches, optimizing outcomes and enhancing quality of life in Chiari malformation management.

Printed in Dunstable, United Kingdom